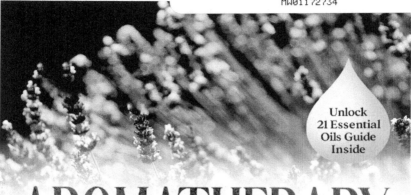

Unlock
21 Essential
Oils Guide
Inside

AROMATHERAPY

FOR SELF CARE

ESSENTIAL OILS FOR WOMEN
The Key to Natural Wellness, Beauty
Care and Emotional Well-Being

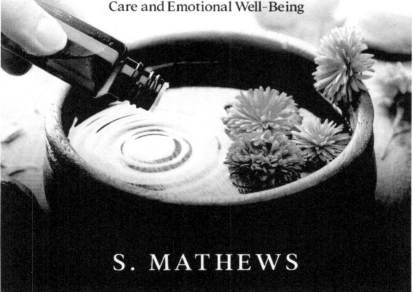

S. MATHEWS

AROMATHERAPY FOR SELF-CARE

ESSENTIAL OILS FOR WOMEN: THE KEY TO NATURAL WELLNESS, STRESS RELIEF, BEAUTY CARE, AND EMOTIONAL WELL-BEING

S. MATHEWS

TABLE OF CONTENTS

INTRODUCTION

In a world where everyday women and glamorous actresses alike seek the secrets of serenity and the allure of natural beauty, the captivating journey into the world of essential oils begins.

Katie Couric, the captivating journalist, finds calm and comfort in lavender and chamomile oils, whisking away stress and embracing tranquility. Meanwhile, Victoria Beckham, the fashion forward-icon, incorporates geranium oil into her beauty routine to promote a healthy and radiant complexion. *(firstforwomen.com)*

Transform your life with the fantastic advantages of essential oils. Uncover peppermint oil's refreshing and stimulating impacts that can enliven your senses and refresh your thoughts. Discover how a mere sniff of eucalyptus oil can effortlessly clear your sinuses, breathing a fresh wave of vitality into your wellness routine. Get ready to unlock the secrets concealed within these tiny vials and tap into the remarkable potential of essential oils to rejuvenate your body, mind, and spirit.

Step into an insightful journey within the pages of this book which aims to teach women and mothers all they need to know about aromatherapy for self-care and the many benefits essential oils can have in their daily lives.

Are you an essential oil enthusiast? If not yet, I predict that you will be soon! The global market for essential oils has been growing at a staggering rate over the past few years. Statista estimated the value of the essential oils market to be around $17 billion in 2017, and it's projected to reach a whopping $27 billion by 2022 (Petruzzi, 2022). That's an astonishing increase of $10 billion in merely five years! And if you thought this trend was only popular in one region, think again. While Europe currently leads the pack, North America and the Asia Pacific region are hot on its heels.

Carla, a woman and mother of two busy toddlers, had been feeling more anxious than usual lately. Between her hectic work schedule and family responsibilities, she never seemed to find a moment to relax.

She heard about the benefits of aromatherapy for reducing stress and decided to try it. Carla then started researching different essential oils and their properties. Lavender, bergamot, and frankincense were generally recommended for relaxation and stress reduction. Carla decided to try them all.

She purchased a diffuser and started using it before bedtime. She also infused her bath water with drops of essential oils. She even started carrying a rollerball of frankincense oil with her and applying it to her wrists and temples whenever she felt stressed.

As time passed, Carla noticed a significant improvement in her overall mood and stress levels. She felt more relaxed and centered during hectic workdays or family gatherings. So she started recommending essential oils to her friends and family, who were also looking for natural ways to reduce stress.

Carla was amazed at how such a simple and natural solution could make such a big difference in her life. Her success with aromatherapy inspired her. She joined an essential oil group on social media and started sharing ideas with others with a mutual interest in essential oils. Through this community, she learned about the extraction and manufacturing processes and how to ensure that the essential oils she used were of the highest quality.

Carla's experience with essential oils is a testimony to the power of aromatherapy. By taking the time to research and experiment with different oils, she found a natural and effective solution to her anxiety. With the help of a supportive community and high-quality oils, she was able to improve her overall well-being and live a more balanced life.

The use of essential oils for their potential health benefits has gained significant attention in recent years. Even celebrities like Kerry Washington and Ellen Pompeo are reportedly fans of essential oil use (Anglis, 2019).

Kerry Washington uses a homemade scalp tonic as part of her hair-care routine. The tonic is a DIY (Do it Yourself) mixture she puts together and applies to her scalp using a spray bottle. The components of her homemade scalp tonic include distilled water as the base ingredient, providing hydration to the scalp, and non-alcohol witch hazel to keep the skin on the scalp fresh and clean. Kerry Washington incorporates several essential oils into her scalp tonic for their beneficial properties. Among the essential oils discussed, rosemary is noted for its ability to promote hair growth and enhance scalp health; eucalyptus for its refreshing and invigorating anti-inflammatory properties; and peppermint oil, which provides a cooling sensation and can help soothe an itchy scalp. Some say it helps with hair growth. Last but not least, it also contains lavender essential oil, which is generally used for its calming and relaxing properties and antimicrobial effects, which are beneficial for maintaining scalp health.

According to Kerry, her homemade scalp tonic serves multiple purposes. It helps keep the scalp healthy, prevents itchiness, and addresses product buildup when wearing protective styles like braids for a prolonged period (Wohlner, 2020).

In the initial phases of her acting journey, Ellen Pompeo, a prominent figure in the entertainment industry, had her favored fragrances, which encompassed Kai perfume and Michael Kors' Island Fiji. However, her approach to personal care changed after becoming a mother, as she embraced clean living by eliminating parabens, sulfates, and other undesirable ingredients from her household (Ellis, 2022).

To maintain a fresh scent, Ellen opted for essential oils instead of mainstream perfumes. Surprisingly, she turned to Whole Foods for her essential oil needs. Her preferred aromatic choices include citrus, sandalwood, geranium, and rose. She creates a blend of these oils with alkaline water, resulting in a refreshing mist that she sprays on for a revitalizing experience.

Considering her constant exposure to crowds as an actress, Ellen understands the importance of smelling pleasant throughout the day. Despite not being particularly fond of perfume, she has relied on natural alternatives for the past 25 years to ensure she smells good while being mindful of the environment and her skin (Ellis, 2022).

Guided by the insights and experiences of these celebrities, we embark into the journey of aromatherapy. Aromatherapy utilizes concentrated plant extracts, known as essential oils, to support emotional and physical wellness.

- Essential oils offer aromatic and therapeutic properties for relaxation, stress relief, improved health, and overall health support.
- Different essential oils have unique benefits, like lavender for relaxation or peppermint for mental clarity.
- Aromatherapy can be carried out in different ways, such as inhaling, applying topically, and diffusing.
- Incorporating aromatherapy into daily routines can be done with diffusers, massage oils, bath additives, or inhalation techniques.

- Aromatherapy complements conventional medical treatments, enhancing well-being and promoting balance and harmony (NCCIH: Aromatherapy, 2020).

This book offers guidance on utilizing essential oils for women, children, and the whole family in addressing common ailments, promoting calmness, and enhancing better sleep quality.

People have used essential oils for their therapeutic and medicinal properties for centuries. These oils are concentrated aromatic compounds extracted from plants. Essential oils are derived from different plant components, such as bark, flowers, leaves, stems, and roots. The essential oils used for aromatherapy are obtained using distillation or cold-pressing methods to extract their volatile components (NCCIH: Aromatherapy, 2020).

Let's take a sneak peek into the existence of essential oils. It is believed to have been used for the first time by the ancient Egyptians approximately 3,500 years ago (Nervik, 2021). Essential oils have been used in traditional medicine practices like herbalism, ayurveda, and traditional Chinese medicine for centuries. These items were appreciated for improving people's physical, mental, and emotional well-being (*NCCIH: Aromatherapy*, 2020). Over time, essential oils gained popularity in other fields, including perfumery, cosmetics, and the culinary arts.

While scientific research on essential oils is ongoing, some studies suggest that certain oils possess anti-inflammatory, antioxidant, and antimicrobial properties. For example, tea tree oil has been investigated for its antimicrobial activity against various pathogens (Carson et al., 2006), while lavender oil has been studied for its potential calming and sleep-inducing effects (Buchbauer et al., 2011). The benefits of tea tree and lavender oils are a few examples that show the potential that lies within the power of essential oils, offering a natural path to wellness and rejuvenation.

In *Aromatherapy for Self-Care*, we'll delve deeper into the following topics:

- Aromatherapy Archives—All About Oils
- The Art of Mastering Essential Oils—Knowing Your Oils
- Essential Oils Unveiled—How to Use Oils
- The Essential Oil Health Guide
- Beyond the After-Shave—Oils for Men
- The Mother's Guide to Essential Oils
- Finding the Perfect Blend for Your Child's Age
- Toxic to Tranquil—Transform Your Home with Essential Oils
- Your Fragrance Swatches

As a woman and a mother of three, I know firsthand the challenges of balancing life, motherhood, work, and self-care. I have also struggled with stress, anxiety, and sleep issues and have constantly searched for ways to improve my health and well-being.

During my uphill journey, I discovered the power of essential oils. Eventually, I began experimenting with different blends and applications and was amazed at how effectively they reduced stress, improved sleep quality, and promoted relaxation. Essential oils soon became a permanent part of our household and lifestyle. I discovered the remarkable soothing properties of lavender oil when my children had cuts or bruises. I gently applied lavender oil diluted with a carrier oil and gently applied on the area. The soothing aroma and anti-inflammatory properties of lavender oil helped promote quick relief. Eucalyptus oil also has been a trusted companion in times of congestion. A few drops with a carrier oil applied on the chest, or diffused in the air, help with stuffy noses and helps ease breathing.

Inspired by my experiences, I wrote Aromatherapy for Self-Care to share my knowledge and insights with other busy women and mothers. Through my book, I hope to empower other women to take control of their health and wellness by using essential oils safely and effectively.

As someone who has been there myself, I understand the unique needs and concerns of a busy schedule. In this book, I aim to provide you with practical, accessible advice and more that is easy to implement in everyday life. Whether you're a seasoned essential oil user or new to the world of aromatherapy, Aromatherapy for Self-Care is a must-read for any woman looking to prioritize their health and well-being and also for every mother who needs a little bit of extra help around the house.

Within the pages of this book, you'll learn more about the many benefits you will gain by using essential oils, such as:

- Relaxation and stress relief: Many essential oils possess calming properties that aid in reducing anxiety and stress and promote relaxation. Lavender, chamomile, and bergamot are a few examples of oils known for their soothing effects.
- Improved sleep: Lavender and vetiver are essential oils that enhance sleep quality. Diffusing these oils or adding a few drops to a bath or on your pillow can create a relaxing environment that aids in falling asleep faster and improving sleep quality.
- Mood enhancement: Essential oils can positively impact mood and emotions. Citrus oils like orange, lemon, and grapefruit are known for their uplifting properties, while oils like ylang-ylang and clary sage can promote joy and calmness.
- Boosted energy and focus: Peppermint and rosemary, for example, have stimulating qualities that can boost alertness, concentration, and energy levels. Inhalation or topical application of these oils may help combat fatigue and improve mental clarity.
- Natural skincare: To improve your skin, consider using essential oils in your skincare routine. Lavender, tea tree, and chamomile oils have properties that can soothe and protect your skin. It's important to dilute the oils correctly and perform a patch test beforehand to make sure they are compatible with your skin type.
- Pain relief: Certain essential oils, such as eucalyptus and peppermint, have analgesic properties and may relieve headaches, muscle aches, and joint pain. You can apply

diluted oils topically or use them in massage blends for localized pain management.

- Immune support: Eucalyptus, tea tree, and oregano are examples of essential oils with antimicrobial properties that can assist in bolstering the immune system. Diffusing these oils or using them in cleaning products may help create a healthier environment, especially during cold and flu seasons.
- Emotional support: Essential oils can support emotional well-being by providing comfort and balance. Oils like lavender, frankincense, and geranium are often used in aromatherapy practices to promote emotional stability and uplift moods.
- Bonding and relaxation with children: Using essential oils safely and age-appropriately can create a calming and soothing atmosphere for children. Oils like chamomile, lavender, and mandarin can help promote relaxation, improve sleep, and enhance the bonding experience between mothers and their children.

Join me on this journey of discovering the benefits and secrets of using essential oils for self-care and many other purposes.

Important: Essential oils should be used cautiously and under proper guidance. They are highly concentrated and should be diluted before topical application or ingestion. Individual responses to essential oils can vary; some people may be allergic to or sensitive to certain oils. If you have chronic conditions or are prone to allergies, first discuss the use of oils with your healthcare practitioner.

1

AROMATHERAPY ARCHIVES—ALL ABOUT OILS

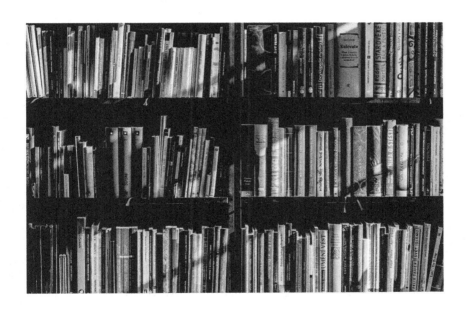

THE ESSENCE OF ESSENTIAL OILS

L et us immerse into the wealth of knowledge and understand the very essence of essential oils. Essential oils are highly concentrated plant extracts that capture various plants' natural compounds and fragrances (essence). These oils are obtained through distillation or cold-pressing, which extracts aromatic and medicinal components from different parts of plants, such as flowers, leaves, bark, stems, or roots (West, 2019).

Let's talk about what it means when we say that manufacturers of essential oils extract essential oils from these plants:

- Steam or water distillation: The essential compounds are effectively extracted and separated by passing hot water or steam through plant material. Steam carries the aromatic molecules, and as it cools down, it condenses into a liquid consisting of water and essential oil components. To acquire pure essential oil, the process involves the separation of the oil from the water.
- Cold pressing: Plant matter is mechanically pressed or squeezed to release essential oils from the plant. A good example is when you squeeze or zest a lemon peel, and you can smell the fresh lemon scent. Because the oil glands in citrus fruits are present in the peel, cold pressing is commonly used to obtain essential oils.

After extracting the active compounds from the plant material, manufacturers mix them with a carrier oil. This practice allows them to produce a larger quantity of product from the same amount of essential oil. As soon as carrier oils are added, the resulting mixture is no longer considered a pure essential oil but rather a blend or diluted form (Johnson, 2019). To ensure you are well-informed about essential oils, here are some key points to keep in mind:

- Composition: Essential oils are made of chemical substances like terpenes, aldehydes, esters, and phenols. Each oil has a distinct composition that adds to its qualities and scent.
- Aromatic properties: The aromas of essential oils are known to be strong and distinct. The fragrance of an essential oil comes from its volatile compounds, which evaporate easily and can be detected by our sense of smell.
- Therapeutic uses: Essential oils have been used in traditional medicine for centuries due to their potential therapeutic benefits. Different oils have varying properties, such as anti-inflammatory, antimicrobial, analgesic, calming, or energizing effects. These properties make essential oils popular in aromatherapy, where they are used to promote physical and emotional well-being.
- Application methods: The good news is that you can use your essential oils in unique ways. They can be inhaled through diffusers, steam inhalation, or added to a soaking bath. Some oils can be applied topically but

must be diluted with a carrier oil to prevent skin irritation. The consumption of essential oils is generally discouraged due to the potential toxicity they may possess.

- Safety considerations: While essential oils can offer benefits, it is essential to use them cautiously. It's important to note that certain oils can cause skin sensitivity or allergic reactions, and some oils should not be used during pregnancy or by people with certain medical conditions. It is crucial to do thorough research, follow recommended dilution ratios, and consult a healthcare professional before using essential oils (West, 2019). The information in this book does not substitute medical advice or consultations with healthcare professionals.

The United States Food and Drug Administration (FDA) does not check essential oils for therapeutic purposes (FDA: Aromatherapy, 2022). Therefore, it's necessary to use them responsibly and rely on reputable sources for information and guidance.

Essential oils are highly concentrated extracts derived from plants renowned for their aromatic characteristics and potential therapeutic advantages. Their diverse range of uses and applications has made them popular in various fields, including natural medicine, skincare, and aromatherapy.

THE HISTORY OF ESSENTIAL OILS

The history of essential oils spans thousands of years and encompasses various civilizations and cultures worldwide. Essential oils have been used for their therapeutic and aromatic properties since ancient times. If we could approach our forefathers and ask who first used essential oils for self-care, I bet it would result in quite an argument. Although it's not easy to identify exactly who, when, and where essential oils were first used for therapeutic purposes, we can give you a brief overview of what we know about the history of essential oils in different regions.

- Egypt: Egyptian civilization is known to have a rich history with essential oils. The Egyptians were pioneers in aromatic oils and used them for medicinal, cosmetic, and spiritual purposes. Essential oils were obtained from cedarwood, frankincense, myrrh, and rosemary plants through the extraction process. Essential oils were used in embalming practices, religious ceremonies, and as offerings to the gods.
- China: In China, the use of essential oils can be traced back to around 2697 BCE. Traditional Chinese medicine places considerable importance on aromatic herbs and oils. The Chinese utilized oils such as cinnamon, ginger, and peppermint for their healing properties. Essential oils were integrated into acupuncture, massage, and herbal remedies to promote well-being and balance the body's energy.

- India: Essential oils have a long history in India, where they were used in Ayurvedic medicine. Ayurveda, a traditional Indian system of medicine, incorporates aromatic oils for their therapeutic effects. Oils such as sandalwood, turmeric, and patchouli were generally used in Ayurvedic practices.
- Greece: Greek civilization contributed significantly to developing and understanding essential oils. The renowned physician Hippocrates, considered the father of medicine, used aromatic oils for their healing properties. The Greeks extracted oils from plants like lavender, rosemary, and thyme. These oils were used for their antiseptic, analgesic, and anti-inflammatory properties, as well as for perfumery purposes.
- Rome: The Romans inherited much of their knowledge of essential oils from the Greeks. They used aromatic oils for their hygiene and therapeutic benefits. Essential oils were used in baths, massages, and perfumes. The Romans valued oils like lavender, chamomile, and rose for their calming and soothing properties.
- Persia: Persia (modern-day Iran) played a crucial role in preserving and developing essential oils. This was also the origin of the physician Avicenna. He wrote hundreds of books about different plants and their bodily effects. In his book, The Canon of Medicine, the Persian physician Avicenna documented the distillation process for extracting essential oils. Persian culture embraced aromatic oils for perfumes, massages, and medicinal purposes.

- Europe: During the Middle Ages, essential oils continued to be used in Europe, primarily for their aromatic properties. The practice of distillation became widespread, allowing for the production of essential oils on a larger scale. Popular oils included lavender, bergamot, and rose. Essential oils were used in various applications, including perfumery, herbal remedies, and personal care (Morgan, 2015).

Throughout the centuries, essential oils have evolved and gained recognition for their therapeutic properties. They are now widely used in aromatherapy, natural skincare products, and holistic self-care practices all over the world. These civilizations' historical contributions laid the groundwork for the continued use and exploration of essential oils.

THE SCIENCE BEHIND ESSENTIAL OILS: HOW THEY WORK AND WHAT MAKES THEM EFFECTIVE

Have you ever considered using essential oils for nausea or improving sleep? Your friend recommends peppermint lotion for nausea, while your coworker swears by lavender oil on their pillow. However, it's important to understand whether scientific evidence supports these claims. Do essential oils really work? It seems like everyone these days is recommending aromatherapy. With the essential oils market worth around one billion, it's natural to wonder if these products work (Stierwalt, 2020).

As part of the National Institute of Health, the US National Library of Medicine offers a comprehensive summary of research on the effectiveness of essential oils (Essential Oils, n.d.). At present, there is no scientific research to support the use of essential oils for aromatherapy in curing illnesses. The effects of essential oils as mood elevators or stress relievers are still uncertain and inconclusive, according to research. Some possible benefits are still being studied (*Essential Oils*, n.d.).

While essential oils cannot cure dementia, studies have found that certain oils have been shown to delay the onset of symptoms (Ballard, 2002; Watson, 2018). Lemon and lavender oils have shown promise in reducing agitation and aggression in dementia patients, according to research by Watson (2018) and Ballard (2002). Rosemary oil may enhance memory alertness and quality, while bergamot oil has a calming effect, and peppermint and frankincense oils may improve memory.

Other success stories prove the effectiveness of essential oils. For instance, tea tree oil can treat acne, while oils like thyme, lavender, cedarwood, and rosemary can help with alopecia areata or hair loss (Hay, 1998; Enshaieh, 2007).

Josh, a young man who struggled with acne, had great success using tea tree oil as a natural remedy. He tried different over-the-counter products with little improvement before exploring other options. He applied tea tree oil to his acne-prone skin after mixing it with a carrier oil. Gradually, he saw a reduction in the frequency and severity of breakouts. The properties of tea tree oil work well as an antibacterial and anti-inflammatory agent, which can help soothe the skin, reduce redness, and promote a clearer complexion. This success story highlights the potential of essential oils, like tea tree oil, as effective alternatives for managing acne.

The potential of using essential oils in citrus fruits is fascinating, given their innate ability to fight bacteria naturally. The beneficial effects of combining citrus oil with dead sea salts are the inhibition of bacterial growth in mice and its anti-inflammatory properties (Mizrahi et al., 2006). Did you know that using bergamot, a citrus essential oil, can help prevent causes of food poisoning such as E. coli, listeria, and staphylococcus? (Fisher and Phillips, 2006) Despite numerous studies, clinical trials for essential oils still need to be improved. Therefore, further research is necessary before physicians can prescribe them.

Essential oils have gained much attention from the public due to their potential to address health issues such as migraines, anxiety, stress, insomnia, and memory problems. They are also a good option if you want control over what you put in your medicine cabinet without a prescription. Therefore, conducting further research to explore the remarkable benefits of essential oils is a path worth considering for women seeking a more natural solution to wellness.

Using essential oils has very few reported side effects. However, you should note that lavender and tea tree oils have estrogen-like effects that could lead to breast enlargement in prepubescent boys if applied over a long period of time. This is an exception to the otherwise safe use of these oils. Another thing to consider is that the method of use may determine the safety of the oil.

If you're looking to alleviate stress-related symptoms, consider adding a few drops of essential oils to a warm and soothing bath. This simple self-care action can provide a relaxing escape to your day, leaving you feeling refreshed.

THE POTENCY OF ESSENTIAL OILS

Essential oils are pretty powerful stuff, packed with all sorts of natural goodness. But it's important to be careful with them and dilute them properly so that our bodies can handle them safely. The oils sold in bottles are much more concentrated than those naturally found in the plant, usually 50 to 100 times stronger. It is important to note that absorbing or ingesting essential oils can be dangerous, despite certain websites promoting it. Applying pure essential oils directly to the skin should also be avoided, as their high concentration can cause irritation or chemical burns. Instead, they should be diluted into a blending oil or lotion. It is not recommended that you mix essential oils with water and consume them or give them to your child to consume (Buerger, 2019). The ingestion of essential oils can pose potential risks; further inquiries should be addressed to a qualified healthcare professional.

A popular method of utilizing oils is through a diffuser, but it's important to note that not all diffusers are of the same quality. For those who are new to diffusers, it is recommended to opt for ultrasonic ones. These diffusers release a mist composed of essential oils and water into the air. Once you have more experience with essential oils, you should consider nebulizing diffusers, as they disperse pure, undiluted oil through air mechanisms. It is essential to have a thorough knowledge of the oils you are using, especially if they are undiluted. Here's a helpful tip: It's best to keep your diffuser on for only part of the day. For optimal performance, a high-quality diffuser should be capable of spreading fragrance throughout a room within 30 minutes. Overexposure to some oils, especially when inhaled, can lead to side effects like headaches and an increased heart rate.

It is important to keep oils out of the reach of children and babies, as they can be more sensitive to their potentially harmful effects. Pregnant women should be cautious when using certain oils, as peppermint oil, in particular, is known for its strong ability to induce early labor.

If you want to try using essential oils, it is also valuable if you can consult a certified aromatherapist. These professionals have completed extensive coursework and can provide personalized guidance based on your medical history and the specific properties of the plants.

If you're new to exploring essential oils, you may need clarification on the technical terms used by professional herbalists and natural product crafters. To help you get started safely and confidently, we've put together some straightforward guidelines and tools. These will make it easier for you to understand the basics without feeling overwhelmed.

Essential Oil Dilution Ratios

To use essential oils safely, it's important to dilute them. This is true whether you're using the oils on their own (in a neutral carrier oil) or incorporating them into a finished product like lotion, massage oil, or aroma spray. It's important to use caution when dealing with essential oils due to their high concentration. Regardless of the dilution method you choose, it's important to ensure that the essential oil content makes up only 0.5% to 2% of the entire blend. To achieve the desired result, it is recommended to add 3 to 12 drops of the product per ounce of the final mixture (Christine, 2019).

Perfume Dilutions

To ensure the best results for both you and your child's body care products, it's advised that you use essential oils in a maximum concentration of 2% of your final product volume. When formulating skincare products like creams, lotions, and serums, it's important to consider that they are typically applied generously over large areas of the body. While the product's main purpose, such as moisturizing or smoothing, is typically the primary focus, fragrance remains a crucial aspect. Essential oil-based perfumes offer a unique opportunity to showcase your aroma blends. Since these mixtures are applied in small amounts to specific areas, you may confidently opt to use a higher proportion, up to 5%, to get the desired smell (Christine, 2019).

Helpful Ideas for Diluting Your Oils

- Use the appropriate measuring instruments and ensure precise conversion between various units of measurement.
- It's important to note that not all essential oils have the same potency. Essential oils made from the bark of cinnamon are more aromatic and have a higher potency than those made from cinnamon leaves. To ensure that you get the desired results, it's essential to research the nature of the oils you plan to use, especially when creating your own recipes.
- It's important to choose essential oils that are suitable for the purpose of your recipe. Some oils may not react well to sunlight, so they should be avoided when making a hair serum. It is advisable to familiarize yourself with the properties of the essential oils you intend to use.

Calconic has developed a calculator for dilutions, which you can visit on their website (www.calconic.com). This serves as a valuable tool for essential oil enthusiasts, providing exact measurements and safe guidelines.

Statement of purity: It is important for essential oil labeling to clearly state that the contents of the bottle are 100% pure essential oil. Any absence of this notification could suggest that the oil is a synthetic blend or fragrance oil (Quality & Grades of Essential Oils, 2020).

THE GRADING OF ESSENTIAL OILS

Grading systems for essential oils vary, and there is no universal standard. Here are the primary grades generally used:

- Synthetic: chemically produced oils that mimic natural aromas but lack therapeutic properties.
- Fragrance grade: used for aroma in cosmetics, perfumes, and candles, not for therapeutic use.
- Therapeutic grade: not regulated, used by companies to imply high quality; research specific standards.
- Floral water: a byproduct of steam distillation used in scented products; synthetic or altered versions can have adverse effects.

When purchasing essential oils, choose reputable brands that are transparent about sourcing, production methods, and third-party testing. Consult a qualified professional for safe and effective use if you have specific therapeutic needs.

How to Ensure That You Use High-Quality Essential Oils

How can you check the quality of essential oils without relying on a flawed grading system? I have some valuable tips to share (Martinez, 2022):

- Testing: When buying essential oils, it's important to ensure the company provides GC/MS tests for every batch of oil they sell. Make sure that the tests are evaluated by a qualified professional, such as an aromatherapist or essential oil chemist.

- Labeling: When purchasing essential oils, both the common name (such as Cajeput) and the botanical name (such as Melaleuca cajuputi) should be listed on the label. The label should include safety information specific to that particular oil. To ensure the quality of your essential oils, opt for those certified by either Ecocert or the USDA. Look for labels that indicate the botanical name of the plant, its place of origin (such as South Africa, Australia, or France), the extraction method used (cold-pressing for citrus rinds or steam distillation), and the specific part of the plant from which the oil was extracted, for example, the leaves, roots, or flowers (Galper & Shutes, 2020).

- Features: If you want to ensure that the sandalwood oil you bought is genuine, it should have the usual appearance, fragrance, and texture of other essential oils in its category. Normally, sandalwood oil is very dense, so if the oil you bought is watery and thin, it may not be authentic sandalwood oil.

- Purity: After gaining experience with pure oils, it becomes easier to distinguish if an oil has synthetic additives. It is important to note that most body sprays, candles, and home fragrances contain synthetic ingredients. To determine which essential oils are genuine, you can compare them with one of these products.

- Longevity: When choosing an essential oil company, it's important to consider its longevity in the business. Companies that have been operating for 10+ years generally have greater experience sourcing quality oils.

However, it's worth noting that newer companies shouldn't necessarily be disregarded.

HOW ARE ESSENTIAL OILS REGULATED?

Unlike prescription drugs, essential oils are not regulated by the FDA as pharmaceuticals. According to Anderson (2020), essential oils have not undergone the same level of research as FDA-regulated medications. This means that they are not FDA-approved, but they should still meet FDA compliance standards (Tomaino, n.d.). Although they're not classified as regulated drugs, essential oils can be harmful if misused. Therefore, using them responsibly and storing them safely, away from children, is crucial. It's important to exercise caution when you're using essential oils. Before starting any form of treatment, holistic or otherwise, for a medical ailment, it is crucial that you consult with a licensed and credentialed medical professional.

Cosmetics or drugs—does it matter? Determining whether essential oils are considered cosmetics or drugs can affect their regulation. The distinction between cosmetics and drugs is important because the regulations and requirements for each category differ. The FDA defines cosmetics as products used for cleaning, enhancing beauty, improving attractiveness, or changing appearance when applied to the body (Is It a Cosmetic, a Drug, or Both? (or Is It Soap?), 2022). On the other hand, drugs are intended to diagnose, cure, mitigate, treat, or prevent diseases.

One example is cumin oil, which can cause skin blistering. Some citrus oils can be harmful in cosmetics, mainly when applied to sun-exposed skin. Lemon essential oil is another example of a citrus oil that can cause skin sensitivity when exposed to sunlight. It's important to use caution and limit outside sun exposure or wear protective clothing if using citrus oils.

If essential oils are marketed for cosmetic purposes, they are subject to cosmetic regulations. However, if they are marketed with claims of treating or preventing diseases, they may be classified as drugs and must comply with drug regulations, which involve more stringent requirements. The classification depends on the intended use and claims made by the manufacturer or distributor. The following points are important:

- Who governs advertising claims: The advertising claims made about essential oils are governed by various regulatory bodies depending on the country. In the United States, the FDA oversees essential oils' regulation and advertising claims. The FDA requires that any claims about essential oils' benefits or therapeutic properties be supported by scientific evidence and comply with specific labeling requirements. Misleading or false claims can lead to regulatory action or legal consequences.
- Regulations worldwide: Regulations regarding essential oils vary from country to country. Different countries have different regulatory bodies responsible for overseeing the safety, labeling, and advertising claims related to essential oils. As an illustration, essential oils in the United States are subject to regulation by the

FDA. Similarly, in Europe, the European Medicines Agency (EMA) and European Food Safety Authority (EFSA) hold pivotal responsibilities in overseeing essential oils and their applications (The Regulatory Landscape of Essential Oil Manufacturing Navigating FDA and International Regulations, 2023). Manufacturers, distributors, and consumers need to be aware of the specific regulations in their respective countries to ensure compliance and safety.

- What impacts the quality:
- Plants: The quality of essential oils is influenced by the plants from which they are extracted. Factors such as species, variety, geographic origin, cultivation practices, and harvesting methods can all affect the quality of the oil. Plants grown in optimal conditions and harvested at the right time tend to yield higher-quality essential oils.
- Processing: The methods used to extract essential oils can impact their quality. Different extraction techniques, like cold pressing, steam distillation, or solvent extraction, can yield oils with varying chemical compositions and therapeutic properties. Proper processing techniques, including temperature control and duration, are essential to preserving the integrity of the oil and its beneficial components.
- Packaging and handling: The way essential oils are packaged and handled can also influence their quality. Oils are sensitive to light, air, and heat, which can cause oxidation and degradation of their chemical constituents. High-quality oils are typically packaged in

dark glass bottles with airtight caps to protect them from exposure to external factors that can compromise their quality.

- Storage: Proper storage conditions are crucial for maintaining the quality of essential oils. They should be stored in a dry, cool place, hidden from direct sunlight and heat. Exposure to extreme temperatures can lead to evaporation or degradation of the volatile compounds in the oil, reducing its potency and therapeutic effectiveness.

Ensuring high-quality essential oils involves attention to all these factors, from the selection of plants to the final oil storage, to maintain their therapeutic properties and safety. If you do not live in the United States, you should make sure that you obtain information about regulations in your specific country.

HOW TO KEEP ESSENTIAL OILS SAFE

Essential oils usually last between one and three years after they are made. The shelf life can differ depending on the type of oil, with citrus oils lasting around 6 to 12 months. Essential oils need to be stored in the right way to maintain their quality and make them last longer. Keep them in a cool, dark place in their initial bottles or murky glass containers that are firmly sealed. Expired oils may have reduced potency and therapeutic benefits, and using them could lead to undesirable results or potential skin irritation. Purchase high-quality, pure oils from reputable sources that provide production dates and offer products in dark glass bottles for optimal preservation. Essential oils can be used safely and effectively as long as you pay attention to expiration dates.

HOW TO KEEP ESSENTIAL OILS FRESH FOR LONGER

To maintain their quality and potency, essential oils need to be preserved and utilized in the right way. Here are some basic tips:

- Store oils in a dark and cool place to protect them from light and heat.
- Ensure bottles are tightly sealed to minimize oxygen exposure.
- Avoid moisture and humidity, keeping oils away from areas prone to water contact.
- Use clean tools and avoid contamination during use.
- Consider refrigeration for oils with shorter lifespans, but be cautious of condensation.
- Label and date oils to track their shelf life.
- Purchase oils from reputable sources that store and handle them properly.

Discard any oils that smell off, have changed color or consistency, or cause skin irritation. Follow the expiration date or general shelf-life guidelines provided by the manufacturer to ensure optimal effectiveness and safety. Essential oils will go bad over time, no matter how well you store them, but you can increase their time in use by facilitating proper care.

THE ULTIMATE GUIDE TO PROPERLY ORGANIZING AND STORING ESSENTIAL OILS

Proper organization and storage of essential oils is an important key factor to ensure and maintain quality, potency, and safety. The chart below shows the essential oil guidelines for creating your own organization system when caring for your oils.

Guidelines and Checklist for Organizing and Storing Essential Oils	
Choose a suitable storage area	• Select a cool, dry, and dark location away from direct sunlight, heat sources, and fluctuating temperatures. • Consider using a dedicated storage box, shelf, or cabinet to organize and protect your essential oils.
Use appropriate bottles	• Essential oils should be kept in dark glass bottles, like amber or cobalt blue, to keep them from breaking down in the light. • Make sure the bottles are firmly sealed to keep the oil fresh and prevent air from getting in.
Labeling and inventory	• Label each bottle with the name of the essential oil and its date of purchase or expiration date. • Create an inventory list to keep track of your essential oil collection, including quantity and purchase dates.
Categorize and arrange	• Group essential oils by type or category for easy access. This can be done based on their aroma, therapeutic properties, or personal choice. • Arrange the bottles alphabetically or based on the frequency of use for quick identification.

Check for fake essential oils	• Inspect the packaging: Look for signs of poor-quality packaging, such as misspellings, unclear labels, or low-quality printing. • Analyze the price: Be cautious of unusually low prices, as pure and high-quality essential oils require proper cultivation and extraction processes. • Examine the scent: Authentic essential oils should have a natural and pure aroma characteristic of the plant. Synthetic oils may have an artificial or chemical smell. • Research the source: Purchase essential oils from reputable and trusted brands or suppliers known for their quality standards and transparency. • Seek third-party testing: Look for essential oil brands that provide batch-specific testing reports from independent laboratories, ensuring purity and authenticity.
Rotate and use oils	• Regularly rotate your oils to ensure they are used within their recommended shelf life. • Follow proper dilution guidelines and usage recommendations for safe and effective application.
Maintain safety precautions	• Safely store essential oils where your children and pets can't reach them. • Use caution during pregnancy, with medical conditions, or if you have sensitivities or allergies.
Perform regular quality checks	• Check the appearance, consistency, and aroma of the essential oils periodically to ensure they have not deteriorated or become rancid. • If an essential oil shows signs of discoloration, cloudiness, or an off smell, it may have degraded and should be discarded.
Essential oil storage checklist	• Store in a cool, dry, and dark location. • Use dark glass bottles and firmly seal them. • On each bottle, write the name of the oil and the date it was made and opened. • Categorize and arrange oils for easy access. • Inspect packaging, price, scent, and source to detect fake oils. • Rotate oils and use them before they go bad. • Follow safety precautions. • Perform regular quality checks.

2

THE ART OF MASTERING ESSENTIAL OILS—KNOWING YOUR OILS

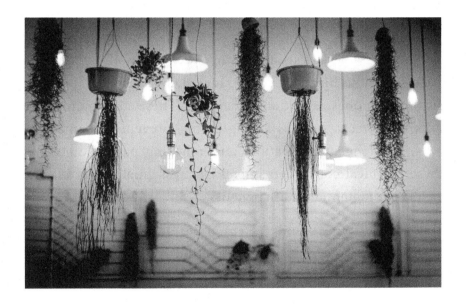

I n chapter one, we talked about how the use of pure essential oils is beneficial over the use of synthetic fragrance oils. Let's discuss in more detail what makes essential oils different and unique from other oils.

Essential oils are distinct and unique from other oils due to their chemical properties, combination of compounds, and organic origin directly from plants.

CHEMICAL COMBINATION AND PROPERTIES OF ESSENTIAL OILS

Essential oils are volatile and highly concentrated liquids composed of a complex mixture of chemical compounds. They are typically extracted from various parts of plants, such as leaves, flowers, stems, bark, or roots. The chemical composition of essential oils can vary widely depending on the plant species, geographical location, climate, and extraction methods.

The chemical properties of essential oils contribute to their unique characteristics and therapeutic effects. Essential oils contain various bioactive compounds such as terpenes, phenols, alcohols, ketones, esters, and aldehydes. These compounds have different effects, such as killing germs, preventing damage to cells, reducing inflammation, and relieving pain. Combining these chemical constituents gives each essential oil its specific aroma and potential health benefits.

Unlike other types of oils, essential oils are not composed of a single compound but a combination of several chemical constituents. This complex mixture of compounds is responsible for the diverse therapeutic properties and unique fragrance associated with each essential oil. One example is lavender essential oil, which has compounds such as linalool and linalyl acetate that can help create a calming and relaxing effect.

The combination of compounds in essential oils also allows for synergistic effects, where the interaction between different constituents enhances their individual therapeutic properties. This synergistic effect can increase the efficacy and broaden the range of applications of essential oils.

ORGANIC ORIGIN DIRECTLY FROM THE PLANT

The organic origin of essential oils is another aspect that sets them apart from other oils. Essential oils can be sourced from organically grown plants, which means they are cultivated without synthetic fertilizers, pesticides, or genetic modification. This organic cultivation ensures that essential oils are considered more natural and environmentally friendly, and free from chemical residues.

Essential oils are extracted from plant materials using specific techniques tailored to the plant part containing the oils. They are not artificially formed in laboratories. These oils are essentially the liquid essence of the plants themselves.

HOW ARE ESSENTIAL OILS MADE?

There are several popular methods employed for extracting essential oils, each with its own advantages and suitability depending on the plant material. Some of these methods are enfleurage, distillation through steam, solvent extracting, CO_2 extracting, cold press harvesting, maceration, and distillation through water (A Comprehensive Guide to Essential Oil Extraction Methods, 2017). These extraction methods ensure that essential oils retain their natural properties and are obtained directly from plant material.

The quality of essential oils can be influenced by the extraction method, which determines the pressure and temperature conditions applied during the process. Different extraction techniques are better suited for specific types of plants and their respective parts. For example, cold press harvesting is better than enfleurage for getting oil out of the peels of citrus fruits. This is because the peels need to be punctured and squeezed, which is not achievable through the enfleurage method.

Here, we'll talk about some of the ways that essential oils are crafted:

- Concretes and absolutes: Absolutes and concretes are forms of aromatic plant products that are very condensed. To make them, plant materials are mixed with a solvent and waxes or resins, heated in a vacuum, and washed with ethyl alcohol. Absolutes are used in perfumery to add rich and complex fragrances like tobacco, oakmoss, jasmine, and rose. They provide depth and character to alcohol-based perfumes (Villafranco, 2018).
- Steam distillation: One of the most common ways to get essential oils from plants is to use steam distillation. Imagine standing in a field of lavender, surrounded by rows of vibrant purple flowers gently swaying in the breeze. In steam distillation, these beautiful lavender blossoms are carefully placed in a distillation apparatus.

As steam moves through the plant material, it picks up the scents from the flowers. The essential oil-carrying steam then condenses, and the resulting lavender essential oil is fragrant and good for you.

- Water distillation: This is a special way to get the oil out of florals like roses and orange blossoms that would stick together during distillation if exposed to steam. Remember the Valentine's Day bouquet of 12 red roses you got? In water distillation, those fragrant roses are immersed in hot water. As the water heats up, steam is produced, carrying the essential oil compounds from the roses. The steam is condensed, and the essential oil and water are separated, leaving behind a captivating rose essential oil that captures the essence of romance and beauty.

- Cold pressing: Imagine strolling through an olive grove with rows of ripe olives hanging from the branches. Cold press extraction, also known as expression, is generally used to obtain essential oils from citrus peels and some other plant materials. In this method, mechanical pressure is applied to the plant material, releasing the essential oil from the peel's glands. The oil is then separated from the fruit juice, resulting in a vibrant and invigorating essential oil.

- Maceration method: Transport yourself to a picturesque garden filled with an abundance of blooming roses. Maceration (or infusion) involves immersing plant material, such as rose petals, in a carrier oil, like almond or jojoba oil. Over time, the aromatic compounds infuse into the carrier oil, creating a scented oil that captures the romantic and intoxicating fragrance of the roses. Unlike distilled oils, macerated oils capture more of the plant's essence as they retain heavier and larger plant molecules. This characteristic allows the oil to retain more of the valuable offerings present in the plant. It is important to note that macerated oil may become cloudy or develop an unpleasant odor if it becomes rancid. As an "active botanical," 5–10% of an oil that has been macerated can be used in making cosmetics. It can also be used in greater quantities to replace plain base oils (A Comprehensive Guide to Essential Oil Extraction Methods, 2017).

- Microwave-assisted extraction (MAE): MAE is a modern method used to retrieve essential oils from plant material. In this method, the plant material is placed in a solvent, and microwave energy is applied. The microwaves generate heat, accelerating the extraction process by facilitating the release of essential oil from the plant material. MAE offers advantages such as shorter extraction times and higher yields compared to traditional methods (Fokou et al., 2020).

- Solvent extraction: Solvent extraction is applied to plants that cannot be effectively processed through steam distillation or cold pressing. Picture yourself walking through a sunny citrus orchard, with the air filled with the tangy scent of ripe oranges. Solvent extraction is often used for citrus fruits, including grapefruits, oranges, limes, and lemons (Davis, 2023). The fruit peels are pressed and mixed with a solvent, such as hexane or ethanol, which dissolves the essential oil. After the mixture is filtered, the solvent evaporates, leaving behind a concentrated citrus essential oil bursting with zesty and refreshing notes.

- Supercritical fluid (CO2) extraction: Imagine strolling through a dense forest, surrounded by towering evergreen trees. CO2 extraction uses carbon dioxide's power to get essential oils out of plants. In this method, CO2 is pressurized until it becomes a liquid, which is then used as a solvent to extract the oils. This process preserves the plants' delicate aroma and therapeutic properties, resulting in high-quality essential oils that capture the essence of the forest.

- Enfleurage: Picture a field of jasmine flowers basking in the warm glow of the sun. Enfleurage is a traditional method that involves placing flower petals on a greased glass plate or fabric. As the flowers wilt, they release their aromatic compounds, which are absorbed by the greasy medium. The process is repeated with fresh flowers until the medium becomes saturated with the desired scent. The greasy medium is then washed with alcohol to extract the essential oil, resulting in a luxurious and floral fragrance.

These extraction methods ensure that essential oils retain their natural properties and are obtained directly from the plant material, allowing us to experience their aromatic wonders in various aspects of our lives.

SAFETY IN ESSENTIAL OILS

Safety is an important consideration when using essential oils, as they are highly concentrated extracts derived from plants and can have potent effects on the body. While essential oils offer many potential benefits, it is crucial to understand the potential risks, side effects, and precautions associated with their use to ensure safe and responsible usage.

- Risks: One of the main risks associated with essential oils is the potential for allergic reactions. Some individuals may develop sensitivities or allergies to specific essential oils, manifesting as skin irritation, redness, itching, or respiratory symptoms. It is necessary to perform a patch test before using a new essential oil topically and to discontinue use if any adverse reactions occur.
- In children: It's generally recommended to use more diluted, smaller amounts of essential oils. Exercise additional caution when selecting oils for use in babies and children, or alternatively, avoid their use altogether. Specific attention should be given to certain essential oils like peppermint, which should not be used with children under the age of six (Halcon, n.d.). Peppermint oil contains menthol, a major chemical component, which has been associated with instances of respiratory arrest in young children and severe jaundice in babies with G6PD, a common genetic enzyme deficiency. To ensure safety, it is crucial to store essential oils in bottles with single-drop dispensers, keeping them out

of the reach of children. Even small amounts, as little as a teaspoon, if accidentally ingested, can have serious health consequences.

- During pregnancy: It is important to exercise caution when using essential oils during pregnancy due to their ability to cross the placental barrier. Limited clinical research is available in this area, highlighting the need for careful consideration. True lavender (Lavandula angustifolia) is a gentle essential oil that midwives sometimes use at the time of the baby's birth process and shortly after, and it has shown positive outcomes (Halcon, n.d.). However, it is important to be cautious when using essential oils during pregnancy, infancy, and early childhood, just as with any other substance. If you have any doubts or concerns, you should seek guidance from a knowledgeable healthcare provider who can provide appropriate advice and recommendations.

- Side effects: While essential oils are generally considered safe when used properly, they can cause side effects in some individuals. Common side effects include skin irritation, allergic reactions, headaches, dizziness, nausea, or respiratory issues. These side effects may vary depending on the individual's sensitivity, the oil concentration, and the application method. Diluting essential oils with a suitable carrier oil and using them in moderation can minimize the risk of side effects.

- Application precautions: Proper application is crucial to ensuring the safe use of essential oils. It is necessary to follow the recommended dilution guidelines from reputable sources and avoid applying undiluted essential oils directly to the skin. Some essential oils may be too potent for direct skin contact and can cause irritation or burns. Essential oils should be kept away from sensitive areas such as the eyes, mucous membranes, or open wounds. When using essential oils for aromatherapy, ensuring proper ventilation and avoiding prolonged exposure to concentrated vapors are vital.

- Skin sensitivity: Skin sensitivity is an important consideration when using essential oils. Specific individuals may have naturally sensitive skin, making them more prone to adverse reactions. It is advisable to perform a patch test on a small part of your skin before administering an essential oil to a bigger area. This involves applying a small amount of diluted oil to the inner forearm and monitoring the area for any signs of irritation or allergic reaction. If irritation occurs, it is best to avoid using that particular oil or to further dilute it before application.

- Phototoxicity: This condition can occur when an essential oil is applied to the skin and placed in contact with the sun. This phenomenon is generally associated with specific citrus oils, including bergamot, lemon, lime, orange, and angelica. To illustrate, if you apply a solution containing orange essential oil to your skin and subsequently expose yourself to sunlight or use a tanning bed, you are likely to experience sunburn or even more severe burns.

- Contact sensitivity: This refers to a diverse reaction that can occur following the use of an essential oil. This reaction typically manifests as an itchy rash or the development of hives. It is important to note that contact sensitivity can occur even after initial contact with an essential oil. The immune system reacts to specific chemicals present in the essential oil, triggering this unpleasant response. Interestingly, the intensity of the reaction may appear disproportionate to the level of exposure. It is worth mentioning that older or modified essential oils have a higher likelihood of causing skin reactions.

- Endocrine system disruptors: The endocrine system regulates vital body functions like metabolism, sleep, mood, and growth. Hormonal imbalances can cause symptoms such as weight gain, mood swings, and disrupted sleep. Some essential oils can disrupt hormone production, affecting development, reproduction, and the immune system. For example, lavender oil has been linked to girls getting breasts early, and both lavender oil and tea tree oil can cause boys to get breast tissue that grows in an abnormal way. To avoid complications, it's better not to use lavender and tea tree oils in children, teenagers, pregnant women, and individuals with hormone-related medical conditions like diabetes. Consult healthcare providers before using essential oils topically or with a diffuser (Capritto, 2020).

The safety of using essential oils depends on your own health, personal choices, and considerations. Factors such as allergy symptoms, sleep quality, the presence of pets, and other household members should be taken into account when making decisions about essential oil usage.

USING ESSENTIAL OILS IN HOSPITAL

Hospital-based aromatherapy programs are becoming increasingly prevalent as healthcare providers recognize the potential benefits of using essential oils in healthcare settings. These programs involve the controlled and supervised use of essential oils to support patients' well-being and complement traditional medical care.

According to the Tisserand Institute, hospital-based aromatherapy programs are designed to enhance patient comfort, manage pain and anxiety, improve sleep, and promote relaxation. These programs typically involve the collaboration of healthcare professionals, including nurses, aromatherapists, and integrative medicine practitioners.

The implementation of aromatherapy in hospitals follows a structured approach, often involving the following steps of a nursing care plan (Pace, 2019):

- Assessment: Healthcare providers assess the patient's medical history, current condition, and specific needs to determine the appropriate essential oils and methods of application.

- Planning: Based on the assessment, a personalized aromatherapy plan is created for the patient, considering factors such as contraindications, personal priorities, and desired outcomes.
- Implementation: The selected essential oils are administered to the patient using various methods of application, depending on the individual's needs and the goals of the treatment.
- Evaluation: The healthcare team continuously monitors and evaluates the patient's response to the aromatherapy interventions, making adjustments as necessary to optimize the outcomes.
- Documentation: Comprehensive documentation of the aromatherapy interventions and their effects on the patient's well-being is an essential part of the care plan.

Various methods of essential oil application can be utilized in hospital settings, depending on the desired therapeutic effects and patient preferences. These methods include:

- Active diffusion: Essential oils are diffused into the air using devices such as nebulizers or diffusers, allowing patients to inhale the aromatic molecules.
- Passive/warming diffusion: Essential oils are added to warm water or heating devices to release their aroma gradually throughout the room, promoting a calming and relaxing environment.
- Personal inhaler: A small, portable inhaler containing a specific essential oil or blend is given to the patient,

allowing them to inhale the aroma as needed for symptom management.
- Aroma patch: A patch infused with essential oils is applied to the patient's clothing or bedding, continuously releasing aromatic molecules throughout the day or night.
- Topical application: In some cases, essential oils may be applied topically in diluted forms for targeted effects, such as massage or localized treatments.

Aromatherapy in hospitals is utilized in a variety of healthcare settings. These may include oncology units, maternity wards, surgical departments, intensive care units (ICUs), and palliative care centers. The specific application of aromatherapy depends on the needs and conditions of the patients in each setting.

Research and evidence supporting the use of aromatherapy in healthcare continue to grow. Studies have shown positive effects of aromatherapy in reducing pain, anxiety, and stress, enhancing sleep quality, and improving overall well-being for patients. However, it is important to note that essential oils should be used under the guidance of trained healthcare professionals to ensure safety, use appropriate dosages, and avoid potential interactions or adverse effects.

ESSENTIAL OILS ACTIVITY

Designing flashcards can be a helpful way to keep important information about essential oils easily accessible. Here are some key details that can be included on the flashcards:

- Oil name: Write the name of the essential oil at the top of the flashcard for quick guidance.
- Botanical name: Include the scientific or botanical name of the essential oil, as it can help ensure accuracy and avoid confusion with similar-sounding oils.
- Aroma description: Describe the aroma of the oil using adjectives such as floral, citrusy, woody, or herbal. This can give users a quick idea of the oil's scent profile.
- Extraction method: Specify the method used to extract the essential oil, such as steam distillation, cold-pressing, or solvent extraction. This information can provide insights into the oil's potency and properties.
- Main benefits: Highlight the primary therapeutic benefits or uses of the oil. For example, if it is known for its calming properties or ability to relieve muscle tension, note that on the flashcard.
- Dilution ratio: Indicate the recommended dilution ratio for safe topical use. This can be expressed as a percentage or the number of drops of carrier oil per drop of essential oil.
- Safety precautions: Include any specific cautions or contraindications for the essential oil. This may include information about skin sensitivity, potential phototoxicity, or precautions for use during pregnancy or with certain medical conditions.
- Blending suggestions: Provide suggestions for oils that pair well with the featured essential oil in aromatherapy blends. This can help users create personalized combinations and enhance the aroma or therapeutic effects.

- Storage instructions: Offer guidance on how to store the essential oil properly to maintain its quality and prolong its shelf life. This may include recommendations for storing in a dark and cool place or using dark glass bottles.
- Additional notes: Leave space for users to jot down any additional information or personal experiences they want to remember about the oil.

For example

Flashcard	
Oil name: lavender	
Botanical name	Lavandula angustifolia
Aroma description	Floral and sweet
Extraction method	Steam distillation
• Main benefits	• Improves mood • Helps with sleep • Improves memory • Relieves pain
Dilution ratio	Blend 5 to 10 drops into a cup of water or carrier oil, like coconut oil, sweet almond oil, or jojoba oil.
Safety precautions	• It is not recommended to swallow lavender essential oil due to its toxicity. • Topical use of lavender oil should be done cautiously, considering individual skin sensitivity. • Further research is needed to establish the safety of lavender during pregnancy and breastfeeding.
Blending suggestions	• Citrus blend: Combine lavender with citrus fruits like lemon, orange, or grapefruit for a refreshing and uplifting aroma. • Herbal blend: Pair lavender with other herbal scents such as rosemary, sage, or mint for a soothing and calming blend. • Floral blend: Mix lavender with floral scents like rose, jasmine, or ylang-ylang for a sweet and romantic fragrance. • Woody blend: Blend lavender with woody aromas like cedarwood, sandalwood, or patchouli for a grounding and earthy scent. • Vanilla blend: Combine lavender with vanilla for a warm and comforting aroma with a touch of sweetness.
Storage instructions	• Keep it in a cool, dark place away from direct sunlight and heat. • Make sure you use only dark glass bottles. Transfer lavender oil to dark glass bottles, such as amber or cobalt blue, as they help protect the oil from light exposure. • Secure the bottle cap tightly to prevent air and moisture from entering, which can lead to oxidation and spoilage of the oil. • Avoid extreme temperature changes. Avoid storing lavender oil in areas with extreme temperature changes, such as near stoves, radiators, or windows. • Ensure that lavender oil is kept in a secure location inaccessible to children and pets.
Additional notes	Before using lavender oil topically, especially if you have sensitive skin, it is advisable to perform a patch test. Apply a small, diluted amount of lavender oil to a small area of skin, like the inner forearm, and wait 24 hours to check for any adverse reactions or allergies.

Flashcard	
Oil name: tea tree	
Botanical name	Melaleuca alternifolia
Aroma description	Medicinal, fresh, and herbaceous
Extraction method	Steam distillation: the leaves of the tea tree plant are heated with steam to release the essential oil.
Main benefits	• Antimicrobial properties make them effective against bacteria, fungi, and viruses. • Used topically for skin conditions, such as acne, fungal infections, cuts, or wounds. • A natural insect repellent. • Potential benefits for respiratory health.
Dilution ratio	The recommended dilution ratio for tea tree oil depends on the specific use and sensitivity of the individual. A common dilution for general topical use is 1–2% tea tree oil in a carrier oil, such as almond or coconut oil. However, for more sensitive areas or specific applications, a lower dilution may be recommended.
Safety precautions	• Ingesting tea tree oil orally should be avoided due to its potential toxicity. • It is meant for external use only and should not be applied to the eyes, inner ears, or sensitive areas without proper dilution. • Some individuals may experience skin irritation or allergic reactions to tea tree oil. It is recommended to perform a patch test before using it extensively. • Ensure that tea tree oil is kept in a secure location inaccessible to children and pets. • If you have any existing medical conditions or are pregnant or breastfeeding, it is advisable to consult a healthcare professional before using tea tree oil.
Blending suggestions	• Tea tree oil blends well with other essential oils such as lavender, peppermint, eucalyptus, lemon, and rosemary. • Refreshing and purifying blend: you can combine tea tree oil with lemon and peppermint. • Soothing and calming blend: tea tree oil can be mixed with lavender and chamomile.

Storage instructions	• Store tea tree oil in a dark and cool place away from direct sunlight and heat sources. • Keep the bottle tightly sealed to prevent oxidation and maintain the oil's potency. • It is recommended to store tea tree oil in amber or dark glass bottles to protect it from UV light. • Avoid storing tea tree oil near volatile substances or chemicals that could potentially react with the oil. • Proper storage helps extend the shelf life of tea tree oil and maintain its effectiveness.
Additional notes	It is important to do a patch test and monitor individual reactions when using tea tree oil or any other essential oil.

Flashcard	
Oil name: bergamot	
Botanical name	Citrus bergamia
Aroma description	Citrusy, fruity, and slightly floral, with a distinctive tangy undertone.
Extraction method	Generally extracted through cold pressing the rinds of the bergamot fruit.
Main benefits	• Its mood-lifting and calming properties are often used in aromatherapy to reduce stress and anxiety and promote relaxation. • Potential antibacterial and antifungal properties. • Used in skincare to help balance oily skin and improve the appearance of blemishes.
Dilution ratio	• The dilution ratio depends on the intended use and individual sensitivity. • For general topical application, a recommended dilution is typically 1–2% bergamot oil in a carrier oil, such as almond oil or jojoba oil. • Adjust the dilution ratio accordingly based on personal choice and guidance from a qualified aromatherapist or healthcare professional.
Safety precautions	• Bergamot oil is photosensitive, which means it can increase the skin's sensitivity to sunlight and UV rays. Avoid direct sunlight or tanning beds for at least 12 hours after applying bergamot oil topically. • Some individuals may experience skin irritation or sensitization when using bergamot oil. It is advisable to perform a patch test before applying it extensively and to discontinue use if any adverse reactions occur. • If you have sensitive skin or are prone to allergies, consult a healthcare professional before using bergamot oil. • Bergamot oil should not be ingested orally unless under the guidance of a qualified healthcare professional. • Ensure that bergamot oil is kept in a secure location inaccessible to children and pets.
Blending suggestions	• Citrus blends: Bergamot oil blends well with other citrus oils such as lemon, lime, and orange, creating a bright and uplifting aroma. • Floral blends: It also complements floral oils like lavender, geranium, and ylang-ylang, adding a citrusy and refreshing note to the blend. • Relaxing blend: combine bergamot oil with lavender and chamomile.

Storage instructions	• Store bergamot oil in a dark and cool place away from direct sunlight and heat sources. • Keep the bottle tightly sealed to prevent oxidation and maintain the oil's freshness. • It is recommended to store bergamot oil in amber or dark glass bottles to protect it from UV light exposure. • Avoid storing bergamot oil near volatile substances or chemicals that could potentially react with the oil. • Proper storage helps preserve the aroma and potency of bergamot oil.
Additional notes	It is important to consider skin sensitivity and perform a patch test before using bergamot oil extensively.

Consider printing the flashcards on sturdy card stock or laminating them to ensure durability. To keep the flashcards organized and easily accessible, you can place them in a wooden tray or box, arranging them alphabetically or by categories based on their properties or benefits.

By understanding essential oils comprehensively, we empower ourselves to make informed decisions when incorporating them into our daily lives. We become better equipped to select oils that align with our individual needs, maximizing their therapeutic benefits.

The next chapter will dive deeper into the practical aspects of using essential oils. We will explore specific application methods, dosage guidelines, and safety considerations. Whether you're new to essential oils or an experienced user, this chapter will equip you with the knowledge and tools necessary to harness the full potential of these oils. Get ready to unlock the secrets of using essential oils effectively and safely to enhance your well-being and promote a healthier lifestyle.

3

ESSENTIAL OILS UNVEILED— HOW TO USE OILS

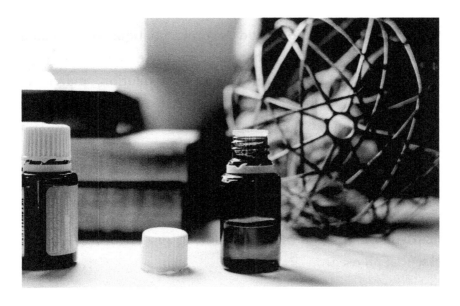

W hen using essential oils, it's important to consider the purpose you have in mind. Essential oils have varying effects, and there is no comprehensive list that clearly defines which oils are helpful for specific health conditions. For example, certain oils like lavender, chamomile, basil, and frankincense are generally known for their calming properties. They may help with anxiety, while bergamot and peppermint oils are considered stimulating and may assist with depression. However, individual responses may vary, so conducting research and consulting with qualified aromatherapists or individuals trained in essential oil use is important. There are community resources and reputable professional organizations that specialize in aromatherapy and essential oils. Examples of a few organizations include the National Association for Holistic Aromatherapy (NAHA) and the International Federation of Professional Aromatherapists (IFPA).

Considering precautions and recommendations when using essential oils is crucial when incorporating them into your routine. Critical factors include proper dilution, individual reactions, and close monitoring for adverse effects. While some tips and examples are provided, it is important that you approach essential oil usage cautiously and ensure you are well-informed about each oil and its specific properties. Remember the designing flashcard activity we did in the previous chapter? Creating flashcards with your priorities and experiences will help you on your journey to achieving successful results with essential oil usage.

If you need help understanding the industry's technical jargon, don't fret. We will provide you with a comprehensive list of carrier oils, explaining everything you need to know in a straightforward and uncomplicated manner.

THE PURPOSE OF CARRIER OILS IN ESSENTIAL OIL USE

If you're curious about the exact meaning of carrier oils, you're at the right place. Carrier oils play an essential role in aromatherapy and blending with essential oils. They are plant-based oils that you can use as a base to dilute essential oils or as a medium to create your own blends, creams, lotions, and massage oils. Carrier oils help provide better consistency to your oils and ensure the safe application of essential oils on your skin or during aromatherapy practices.

Carrier oils are frequently produced by plant fatty portions such as kernels, seeds, or nuts. Some common examples of carrier oils include coconut, almond, jojoba, grapeseed, and olive oils. Each carrier oil has unique properties, such as different textures, absorption rates, and therapeutic benefits.

When blending essential oils with carrier oils, it's important to consider the desired dilution ratio, the specific purpose of the blend, and your specific skin type or sensitivity. Diluting essential oils with carrier oils helps reduce your chances of developing irritated skin because of the increased spreadability and absorption of the blend (Axe, 2022).

Using carrier oils provides a safe and effective way for you to enjoy the benefits of essential oils while ensuring proper application and minimizing the risk of skin irritation.

Selecting the Appropriate Carrier Oil for Your Needs

When selecting the appropriate carrier oils for your needs, understanding their unique properties and benefits is key. Carrier oils do not typically have fragrances, so you can combine them with highly concentrated essential oils. When creating a blend or purchasing a product with a carrier oil base, it's unnecessary to stress over mixing and matching. However, there are a few things to think about. Using carrier oils allows you to apply essential oils to a greater area of your body without applying too much. Using a carrier oil helps minimize the risk of negative skin reactions and ensures adherence to safety guidelines when using essential oils. Are you searching for oils that can help with acne, soothe dry skin, or be the finest massage oils available? It may take some trial and error to discover the ideal oil for your needs.

Let me show you an example of how essential oils can be combined with carrier oils. For optimal results when using tea tree oil to improve the complexion and treat acne on the face, applying more than one to three drops of the topical solution is recommended. This is because these areas, including the chin, nose, forehead, and neck, may require additional coverage. It's essential to note that using the full strength of tea tree oil may not be necessary and can even be too harsh for the desired outcome. If you have skin problems, mix one to three drops of tea tree oil with half a teaspoon of any carrier oil (Axe, 2022). Apply a gentle massage to the affected areas using the mixture.

Have you ever noticed that the scent of lavender or peppermint oil applied to your skin fades away within a few minutes?

The reason for that is that it has been absorbed. The absorption rate slows down when combining carrier oils with essential oils, resulting in a more significant and longer-lasting effect. Carrier oils, which are derived from the fatty portions of plants, do not evaporate as rapidly. Carrier oils are very important if you want your essential oils to last as long as possible.

MOST POPULAR CARRIER OILS

Carrier oils have anti-inflammatory substances, antioxidants, vital fatty acids, and nutrients that are good for the skin. There are a variety of carrier oils with specific benefits and uses (Axe, 2022). Let's start with almond oil and how it can benefit your skincare routine.

Almond Oil

Almond oil is a popular carrier oil due to its antioxidant qualities, which keep the skin soft and healthy. Due to its lightness, almond oil easily penetrates the skin and is often blended with essential oils like tea tree or lavender to gently cleanse the pores and follicles. It has moisturizing qualities that can improve your skin tone and complexion (Axe, 2022).

Usage guidelines

- Make your own shower gel using orange essential oil (Axe, 2022).
- Use it to make under-eye concealer.

- Almond oil is an excellent carrier oil for your diffuser, as it has a light consistency and helps to disperse the fragrance of the essential oils you select.

Now, let's talk about how jojoba oil can help you resolve some of the problems many women experience daily.

Jojoba Oil

Are you struggling with razor burn after shaving? Jojoba oil might be your go-to answer! This plant wax is odorless and works as an emollient carrier oil, making it highly beneficial for skin and hair care.

Jojoba oil has moisturizing and soothing qualities that create a protective barrier on the skin, preventing irritation and discomfort caused by shaving. Its natural antibacterial properties can also prevent infections and ingrown hairs. Because jojoba oil isn't heavy, it's easily absorbed into the skin, reducing friction and providing a calming effect.

Incorporating jojoba oil into your post-shaving routine can help maintain skin health and enhance the overall shaving experience. It's an excellent choice for addressing the concerns of razor burn, allowing you to achieve smoother, more comfortable skin after shaving.

Usage guidelines

- If you have oily skin, using jojoba oil in your homemade moisturizer can help balance the production of oil and prevent a greasy feeling.

- Makeup remover- it's a gentle yet powerful cleanser to take away impurities without stripping the skin's natural oils.
- For those allergic to coconut, jojoba is a versatile substitute ingredient.

Jojoba oil is a great oil to use on your skin for multiple uses. Another carrier oil that's great for skin and hair care is the well-known coconut oil.

Coconut Oil

If you're searching for a carrier oil that works, coconut oil is a great choice. It has a low molecular weight, which means it can penetrate your skin deeply and leave it feeling moisturized. The saturated fats in coconut oil also help to keep your skin smooth and even-toned. It has antiseptic and antimicrobial properties, making it ideal for treating skin conditions like acne, cold sores, and eczema.

Treating dry, rough, itchy, and scaly skin, also known as mild to moderate xerosis, can be done using either virgin coconut oil or mineral oil. A study by Agero and Verallo-Rowell (2004) compared the effectiveness of both options. It involved 34 patients who applied either coconut or mineral oil to their legs twice daily for two weeks (Agero & Verallo-Rowell, 2004). The results showed that both oils were equally effective in improving symptoms of xerosis without causing any adverse effects (Agero & Verallo-Rowell, 2004).

Usage guidelines

- As a carrier oil, coconut oil has numerous applications for the skin.
- To use it, mix one to three drops of any topical essential oil with half a teaspoon of coconut oil and apply the mixture to the area of concern.
- You can create a nourishing full-body moisturizer by combining a few tablespoons of coconut oil with a few drops of your favorite essential oil, such as lavender or rose. Gently massage the mixture onto your skin after a shower, allowing the coconut oil to deeply hydrate and rejuvenate while the aromatic essential oil adds a delightful touch of relaxation. Welcome to the experience of soft and smooth skin that will leave you feeling pampered and refreshed!

Did you think the benefits of olive oil were an old wives' tale? Think again.

Olive Oil

Did you know that natural extra virgin olive oil is good for your heart, brain, and mood, and it can also benefit your skin? It contains healthy fatty acids, anti-inflammatory compounds, and antioxidants that can help hydrate your skin, speed up wound healing, and even fight infections. Olive oil shows potential as a beneficial remedy for skin-related conditions such as seborrheic dermatitis, psoriasis, acne, and atopic dermatitis. Its ability to reduce inflammation and combat bacterial growth contributes to enhancing the overall well-being of your skin. It also has many hair-related benefits, and you may want to try it through scalp massages and deep conditioning treatments to assist with hair health, growth, and even controlling curls that are out of bounds.

Usage guidelines

- You can use olive oil as a DIY hair treatment.
- Hair treatment recipe: Mix 1/4 cup extra-virgin olive oil with 1/2 cup conditioner in a bowl until well blended (yogurt-like consistency). Apply the mixture to your hair and scalp, including the ends. Cover your hair with a shower cap and allow the mixture to remain on for 15 to 30 minutes. Rinse your hair thoroughly and allow it to air dry.

Olive oil has many benefits for your skin and more. Many of us love eating avocado, but did you know how good avocado oil can be for your health, including skin and hair care? Let us delve into it more.

Avocado Oil

If you have dry or rough skin, avocado oil may be a great option. It moisturizes and improves skin texture. Additionally, it can also help remove makeup and hydrate hair. Avocado oil has anti-inflammatory properties and promotes collagen production, making it a useful remedy for treating skin wounds (Axe, 2022).

Usage guidelines

- To utilize avocado oil independently, gently apply a small quantity onto a cotton ball and utilize it to moisturize dry regions on your face, cracked heels, cuticles, and dry hair.
- To make avocado oil a carrier oil, mix one to three droplets of any essential oil that is safe for topical use with half a teaspoon of avocado oil. Rub the combination onto the affected areas (Axe, 2022).

Next, arnica oil is a versatile solution for various skin and body issues, making it one of the best carrier oils for essential oils. Let's find out more.

Arnica Oil

Arnica oil contains helenalin, a powerful anti-inflammatory compound, as well as several fatty acids and thymol, which have been shown to have antibacterial properties.

You can use arnica oil alone to alleviate inflammation, muscle pain, and bruises, or as a potent carrier oil. However, it's essential to check arnica oil products' ingredient labels to ensure they contain a mixture of arnica extracts and base oils, such as olive or almond oil. This dilution is necessary because undiluted arnica oil can irritate the skin.

Do not apply arnica oil to cuts or open wounds. Pregnant or breastfeeding women should refrain from using it since excessive ingestion or application of arnica oil to broken skin can be toxic (Axe, 2022).

Usage guidelines

- To alleviate muscle pain and tension, you can include arnica in a homemade bruise cream.
- Adding relaxing essential oils such as lavender can enhance their soothing properties (Axe, 2022).

Vitamin C is not only found in pills; it actually forms part of the next carrier oil. Now, let's explore the advantages of utilizing rosehip oil as a carrier oil.

Rosehip Oil

Rosehip oil is a carrier oil rich in essential fatty acids that are beneficial for cellular and tissue regeneration. It is also a good source of vitamin C and has anti-aging properties when applied to the skin. It effectively reduces age spots caused by sun damage, improves skin tone and texture, treats eczema, and fights skin infections.

If you have normal to dry skin, rosehip oil is an excellent choice because it is a dry oil that absorbs quickly without leaving an oily residue.

Usage guidelines

- Rosehip oil can be used as a natural moisturizer on its own or mixed with essential oils as a carrier oil, like in the lavender and rose water toner.
- Rose water and lavender toner: In a small bowl, combine four tablespoons rose water, two tablespoons witch hazel, one teaspoon apple cider vinegar, five to ten droplets of rosehip oil, five droplets of tea tree oil, and five droplets of lavender oil (or your preferred essential oil) to make a homemade facial toner. Using a whisk or a spoon, thoroughly combine all ingredients. Fill a small glass spray bottle halfway with the mixture. Close your eyes and spray the toner onto your face after cleansing it. For best results, follow up with your favorite natural facial moisturizer.

Next up, grapefruit seed extract is known for its antimicrobial properties. Let's see how it's used in practice.

Grapefruit Seed Oil

Because it helps fight bacterial, viral, and fungal infections, it is commonly found in personal care products such as wound disinfectant sprays, toothpaste, shower gels, and mouthwashes. Moreover, grapefruit seed extract can be added to your humidifier, laundry, swimming pool, and animal feed to reduce the need for potentially harmful chemicals.

Usage guidelines

- Grapefruit seed oil is an excellent carrier oil for your homemade natural home and body products. It is a natural disinfectant to use to clean household surfaces.
- To make a combination of grapefruit seed extract and essential oil, use equal parts of both. If you want to dilute it more, you can add water or another odorless carrier oil.

Flaxseed Oil

Flaxseed oil has multiple benefits. It can aid digestion, improve heart health, and even help with common skin disorders like eczema. It can also improve skin texture and elasticity when applied topically. This is because it contains a high concentration of omega-3 fatty acids and alpha-linoleic acids, both of which reduce inflammation and promote healthy skin and hair. One of the benefits of using flaxseed oil is that it can help with dry skin by retaining moisture, boosting the healing process of wounds, and giving the skin a radiant look. Its gentle and soothing properties make it an ideal choice for those with sensitive skin.

Usage guidelines

- While flaxseed oil is known for its use in recipes such as smoothies and salads, it can also be applied topically as a carrier oil. Ayurvedic medicine has utilized this oil to balance skin pH, promote wound healing, and remove blemishes.

Now, let's find out why neem oil is a common ingredient in natural skin and beauty products.

Neem Oil

Neem oil's high level of antioxidants protects the skin from damage from the environment. Its lipids and vitamin E are quickly digested into the skin's outer surface, helping to heal cracked or dry skin without making it feel greasy. Neem oil also makes skin more flexible and renews skin cells, which makes it a great ingredient for skin care (Axe, 2022). It is unique among carrier oils in that it acts as a natural insecticide, repelling mosquitoes, flies, and moths.

Usage guidelines

- Neem oil mixed with essential oils like lemon or eucalyptus can be used to treat mosquito bites at home.
- Mix neem oil, jojoba oil, and lavender to make your own wrinkle cream. This cream can be used on your body like a moisturizer (Axe, 2022).

The next oil, derived from the seeds of the evening primrose plant, holds a special place among carrier oils due to its remarkable nourishing properties.

Evening Primrose Oil

Evening primrose oil, similar to other carrier oils, contains a substantial amount of essential lipids. It is used to alleviate skin irritations and enhance skin conditions. Furthermore, the oil possesses anti-inflammatory properties and aids in nerve function and skin elasticity. Although there is no definitive evidence, it has traditionally been utilized to stimulate hair growth (Axe, 2022).

Usage guidelines

- If you're looking to improve your skin's health, balance hormone levels, or treat acne and other skin conditions, try combining evening primrose oil with antimicrobial essential oils like tea tree oil.
- Here's a recipe to promote hair growth: Massage a mixture of evening primrose oil and essential oils such as lavender, cypress, and lemongrass onto your scalp, or add it to your shampoo. (Axe, 2022). Give it a try!

Next up, did you know that magnesium oil is not really an oil? Let's find out why.

Magnesium Oil

It has the texture of oil and is made up of magnesium chloride flakes and water. When applied to the skin, it can aid in muscle relaxation, alleviate fibromyalgia symptoms, and improve skin conditions such as rosacea and acne. It can also help improve blood flow and is a suitable carrier oil for those with oily skin by breaking down fats and oils to prevent an oily appearance.

Usage guidelines

- When you're done in the shower, put magnesium oil and essential oils (such as lavender) in a spray bottle. Then, spray the solution onto your skin (Axe, 2022).

- Blend a muscle-relaxing massage oil or rub with magnesium oil as a carrier (Axe, 2022).
- You can create a magnesium body butter at home, relaxing your muscles and alleviating stress. Replace the jojoba oil with magnesium oil when making the butter (Axe, 2022).

PRECAUTIONS FOR USING CARRIER OILS

Remember that essential oils are highly concentrated substances that must be used correctly and safely in order to reap their benefits while minimizing the risk of adverse reactions. Although most carrier oils are gentle enough for sensitive skin, it is important to check for any allergies or sensitivities.

DILUTING STRONG ESSENTIAL OILS

Remember, essential oils are highly concentrated substances, and using them properly and safely is necessary to enjoy their benefits while minimizing the risk of adverse reactions. When essential oils are too strong, diluting them correctly will ensure safe and effective use. Below are several methods for effectively diluting essential oils:

- Carrier oils: Carrier oils are vegetable oils that can be used to thin essential oils while also nourishing the skin (Axe, 2022). Jojoba oil, coconut oil, almond oil, and grapeseed oil are all popular carrier oils. To make a diluted blend, combine a few drops of essential oil with a tablespoon of carrier oil.

- Unscented lotions or creams: You can also dilute essential oils by adding them to unscented lotions or creams. Mix a few drops of essential oil into a dollop of the lotion or cream before applying it to your skin.
- Bathwater: Essential oils can be diluted in bathwater for a relaxing and aromatic experience. Add a few drops of essential oil to a teaspoon of carrier oil or a cup of Epsom salt before adding it to the bathwater. This helps the oils dissolve in the bathwater.
- Aloe vera gel: Aloe vera gel is another option for dilution, especially if you're dealing with skin irritations. To make a soothing blend, combine a few drops of essential oil with a teaspoon of aloe vera gel.

It's important to note that sensitization can occur when essential oils are used undiluted or in high concentrations. Sensitization refers to developing an allergic reaction or sensitivity to a particular substance. This can manifest as skin irritation, redness, itching, or respiratory symptoms.

To avoid sensitization and ensure the safe use of essential oils, it's crucial to treat them with respect. Here are some guidelines:

- Patch testing: Before using a new essential oil, perform a patch test by applying a small, diluted amount to your inner forearm. Wait for 24 hours to see if any adverse reactions occur. If you experience redness, itching, or irritation, avoiding using that particular oil is best.
- Proper dilution: For topical use, a generally recommended dilution is 2%, which means adding

approximately 12 droplets of essential oil to 1 fluid
ounce (30 ml) of carrier oil or another dilution medium.
This ratio can be adjusted based on individual needs
and the essential oil used.

- Individual sensitivities: Everyone's skin is unique, and
some individuals may be more sensitive to certain
essential oils than others. Pay some attention to what
your body is saying and adjust the dilution ratio or
avoid specific oils if you have adverse reactions.
- Consultation: If you have any underlying health
conditions, are pregnant, or are taking medications, it's
always a good idea to consult a healthcare professional
or a certified aromatherapist before using essential oils.

ESSENTIAL OILS: DILUTION GUIDELINES

I have some helpful guidelines for deciding what ratio of dilution to use in a specific situation:

- 0.25% dilution: This is for children aged three months
to two years. When it comes to using oils on children
under two, aromatherapists tend to prefer hydrosols
over essential oils. Hydrosols will protect younger
children and are tolerated in a mild gentler way to
avoid skin irritation. If used properly, many essential
oils can be safely diffused and applied topically. To
find a list of safe essential oils for children, visit the
MommyPotamus website and search for "safe essential
oils for children" in the top right corner (Dessinger,
2021). A few oils from the list from MommyPotamus

include the following oils: blue tansy, German chamomile, frankincense, lavender, lemon, manuka, patchouli, sandalwood, vanilla. Essential oils should not be applied topically to children under three months old because their skin is more sensitive and permeable to essential oils (Dessinger, 2021). Experts (Tisserand and Young, n.d.) advise caution with infants, as their skin does not mature until three months, and they have a lower metabolic capacity to handle adverse effects. This is especially true for premature babies, and it may be best to avoid all essential oils.

- 1% dilution: If you are looking for a more gentle approach to using essential oils, especially for children aged two to six or for those who are recovering from serious health issues or have a compromised immune system, a 1% dilution is recommended. This dilution is also a good option for pregnant or nursing women, although a dilution of up to 2.5% may also be appropriate. Visit www.mommypotamus.com and search for "safe essential oils pregnancy" to learn more about using essential oils while pregnant or breastfeeding (Dessinger, 2016).
- 1.5% dilution: This is recommended for children ages six through fifteen, but you can rather stick to a 1% dilution. It's hard to measure out half a drop!
- 2% dilution: For most adults, the recommended dilution is typically 2.5%. This is generally used for daily body care products and massage oils. However, for facial skin care, it is better to use a dilution of 1%.

Because it can be difficult to measure half a drop, rounding down to 2% is usually more practical.

- 3–10% dilution: This method is generally employed to provide assistance for specific injuries or sudden illnesses. The appropriate dilution ratio varies based on the circumstances, the person's age, and the type of oil utilized.
- 25% dilution: A 25% dilution of essential oils is not generally used because of their potency. It is, however, used on an occasional basis to help alleviate various issues such as muscle cramps, spasms, and bruising through topical application in combination with a carrier oil.

DILUTION WITH CARRIER OILS TIPS

When figuring out how many drops of carrier oil and essential oil to use in a blend, it's important to think about the density or mixture ratio you want. Here are some tips to help you calculate the number of drops for both oils accurately:

Determine the desired dilution ratio: Decide on the dilution ratio you want to achieve based on the purpose of your blend and the recommended guidelines. Common dilution ratios for topical use range from 1% to 5%, with 2% being a generally used dilution for general purposes.

- Understand the dilution ratio: The dilution ratio refers to the percentage of essential oil in relation to the carrier oil. For example, a 2% dilution means that you'll use two parts of essential oil to 98 parts of carrier oil.

- Calculate the total volume of the blend: Determine the total volume of the blend you want to create. This could be based on the size of the container you're using or the amount you need for a specific application.

- Calculate the volume of carrier oil: Multiply the total volume of the blend by the percentage of carrier oil you want to use. For example, for a 10-milliliter blend at a 2% dilution, you would multiply 10 by 0.98 (98% expressed as a decimal) to get 9.8 milliliters, which represents the volume of carrier oil.

- Calculate the volume of essential oil: Multiply the total volume of the blend by the percentage of essential oil you want to use. Using the same example as above, for a 10-milliliter blend at a 2% dilution, you would multiply 10 by 0.02 (2% expressed as a decimal) to get 0.2 milliliters, which represents the volume of essential oil.

- Convert volume to droplets (drops): Once you have the volume of carrier oil and essential oil, you can estimate the number of droplets using the driblet size of your dropper. Multiply the volume (in ounces) by the estimated number of droplets per ounce to calculate the number of droplets for each oil.

- Adjust based on personal choice and guidelines: If you find a specific number of droplets too strong or weak for your liking, you can adjust the ratio accordingly. Always consider any specific guidelines or safety recommendations for the essential oil you're using.

DILUTION FOR BLENDING TIPS

When it comes to calculating the number of drops of essential oils for blending, it's important to keep in mind that drop sizes can vary depending on the viscosity and size of the dropper. Here are some tips to help you calculate the number of drops or droplets effectively:

- Use a standard dropper: Ideally, a dropper with a standard size will provide you with consistent drop sizes. This will make it easier to calculate and replicate your blends accurately.
- Understand the drop size: Familiarize yourself with the approximate drop size of your dropper. For example, some droppers may produce approximately 20 drops per milliliter, while others may produce around 30 drops per milliliter. Knowing the drop size will help you calculate the desired number of drops more accurately.
- Convert volume to drops: Determine the total volume of carrier oil or blend you want to create. Multiply the volume (in milliliters) by the drop size to estimate the number of drops needed. For instance, if you want to make a 10-milliliter blend and your dropper produces 20 drops per milliliter, you would multiply 10 by 20 to get a total of 200 drops.
- Adjust your drops based on concentration: If you're aiming for a specific concentration, such as a 2% dilution, calculate the number of drops of essential oil accordingly. For example, for a 10-milliliter blend at a

2% dilution, you would multiply 10 by 0.02 (2% expressed as a decimal) to get 0.2. Then, multiply this by the drop size to determine the number of drops needed.

- Start with fewer drops: It's generally recommended to start with fewer drops of essential oil and gradually increase if necessary. This allows you to assess the strength and aroma of the blend before adding more drops.
- Always keep a record: Maintain a record of the number of drops you used for each blend, especially if you find a combination that works well for you. This record will serve as a guide for future blending and help you maintain consistency.

These are general tips, and it's important that you always consider individual sensitivities, specific essential oils, and the purpose of your blend when calculating the number of drops. Adjustments may be necessary.

Application techniques for essential oils involve various methods of using them for therapeutic and aromatic purposes. Here are some generally used application techniques.

APPLICATION TECHNIQUES

Topical Application

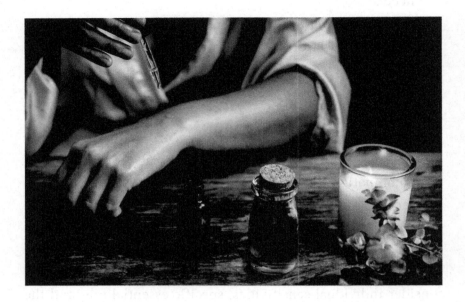

Imagine you are a single woman coming home after a long, exhausting day at work. You deserve some well-deserved self-care to unwind and rejuvenate. Reach for that bottle of lavender essential oil as you enter your sanctuary. Dilute a few droplets with a carrier oil and gently massage the soothing mixture onto your temples and wrists. Let the calming aroma envelop you, easing away the tension and stress of the day. Find solace and tranquility in the comfort of your own home. Topical application is a popular and effective method for using essential oils. It involves applying essential oils directly to the skin, allowing for absorption and localized therapeutic benefits. Here are some specific techniques for topical application:

- Massage: Essential oil massage involves diluting essential oils in a carrier oil and using gentle strokes to apply the blend to the skin. Massaging the oils into the skin not only promotes absorption but also provides relaxation, relieves muscle tension, and supports overall well-being. You can target specific areas or enjoy a full-body massage with essential oils.

- Compresses: Compresses involve using essential oils in combination with warm or cold water to create a soaked cloth or towel that is applied to a specific area of the body. Warm compresses can provide soothing relief for muscle aches, while cold compresses can help reduce inflammation or alleviate discomfort.

- Aromatic bath: Adding essential oils to a bath allows for both inhalation and absorption through the skin. The warm water helps the oils disperse, creating a relaxing and therapeutic environment. Essential oils can be put directly in your bathwater or mixed with a dispersant like Epsom salts or a carrier oil before being added to the bath.

- Epsom salt bath soaks: Epsom salt, also known as magnesium sulfate, can be combined with essential oils to create luxurious and therapeutic bath soaks. Epsom salts help relax muscles, reduce stress, and support detoxification, while essential oils provide aromatic benefits. Simply combine Epsom salts and a few drops of essential oil in a warm bath.

- Foot bath: A foot bath with essential oils can be a rejuvenating and soothing experience. Fill a basin or foot spa with warm water and add a few drops of essential oils. Soak your feet for relaxation, to relieve tiredness, or to promote overall foot health. You can also incorporate Epsom salts for added benefits.

Inhalation

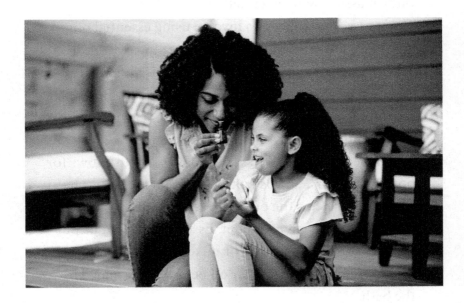

Picture yourself as a dedicated mother determined to start your morning off right, not just for yourself but also for your family. You want an invigorating boost to kickstart your day. Choose a revitalizing blend of citrus essential oils. Add a few drops to a diffuser or a personal inhaler, and breathe in the vibrant aroma that fills the air. Feel your senses awaken as the refreshing scent energizes you. Create an uplifting atmosphere that permeates every corner of your home, setting a positive tone for the day ahead. Inhalation involves breathing in the aroma of essential oils. It can be done in many ways:

- Direct inhalation: To enjoy the aroma of an essential oil, apply a drop or two onto a tissue, cotton ball, or your palms. Cup your hands over your nose and take a deep breath, inhaling the scent.
- Steam inhalation: Add a few drops of essential oil to a bowl of hot water, cover your head with a towel, and inhale the steam. This method is beneficial for respiratory health and relaxation.

Aromatic Diffusion

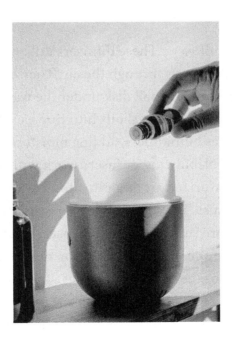

Consider yourself a loving grandmother who desires clarity and wants to overcome momentary brain fog. You understand the power of essential oils and their ability to support mental clarity. Carefully choose a blend known for its clarity-enhancing properties.

Set up a diffuser in your favorite reading corner and fill the air with the gentle fragrance. Breathe in the aroma and feel your mind invigorated, the fog dissipating, and your focus sharpening. Embrace the joy of the present moment and engage in meaningful conversations with your loved ones as you find clarity and renewed mental clarity.

Essential oil diffusers disperse the oils into the air, creating a pleasant and therapeutic atmosphere. There are different types of diffusers available.

- Ultrasonic diffusers: These diffusers utilize water to spread essential oils through the air. They create a fine mist by vibrating a small disk under the water, which breaks down the essential oils into tiny particles. They also double as humidifiers, adding moisture to the air.
- Nebulizers: Nebulizing diffusers work without water and use pressurized air or gas to atomize essential oils into a fine mist. They produce a more concentrated aroma and are suitable for larger spaces. Nebulizers don't alter the chemical composition of the oils, making them ideal for therapeutic purposes.
- Reed diffusers: Reed diffusers consist of a container holding essential oil mixed with a carrier oil. Reeds or sticks are inserted into the liquid, and the oils travel up the reeds, releasing fragrance into the air. They are a simple and low-maintenance option, but the aroma is usually less intense compared to other diffuser types.

When using an ultrasonic diffuser, avoid overfilling or exceeding the maximum water level to ensure proper functioning. Regularly clean your diffuser to prevent oil residue buildup. Read the instruction guide for cleaning and maintenance. This helps maintain the effectiveness of the diffuser and prevents cross-contamination of scents.

Diffusion times may vary depending on the size of the room and personal preference. Start with shorter intervals and adjust as needed to avoid overwhelming or overpowering scents. Some essential oils can be toxic to pets. Ensure that the oils you choose are safe for the specific animals in your household. Don't diffuse if you have pets in the room, and make sure you ventilate the room properly.

Sprays

Imagine a creative woman who loves to personalize her surroundings with delightful scents. She decides to create her own collection of sprays using essential oils, offering a convenient way to enjoy their benefits. With a burst of inspiration, she gathers her favorite oils and sets out to make different types of sprays.

For her home, she creates a refreshing room spray. Diluting a few drops of invigorating citrus essential oils with water, she pours the mixture into a spray bottle. With a quick shake, she spritzes the air, infusing her living space with a revitalizing and uplifting aroma. The spray instantly transforms her home into a sanctuary of freshness and vibrancy.

Next, she crafts a luxurious linen spray for her bedroom. Combining soothing lavender essential oil with distilled water and a touch of witch hazel, she carefully blends the ingredients in a spray bottle. With a gentle mist over her sheets and pillows, the calming scent of lavender envelopes her sleep sanctuary, creating a serene and peaceful ambiance. The spray becomes a part of her nighttime ritual, helping her relax and unwind as she drifts off into a blissful sleep.

Finally, she indulges in creating a refreshing body spray to revitalize herself throughout the day. Mixing her favorite floral and citrus essential oils with a water-alcohol base, she concocts a delightful and energizing fragrance. She fills a small spray bottle and carries it with her wherever she goes. With a few spritzes on her wrists and neck, she uplifts her spirits and feels a renewed sense of confidence and vitality.

Through her creativity and the power of essential oils, she found joy in crafting personalized sprays that enhanced her environment and uplifted her mood.

Creating sprays with essential oils provides a convenient way to enjoy their benefits. You can make various types of sprays, such as room sprays, linen sprays, or refreshing body sprays. These sprays can be made by diluting essential oils with water or a water-alcohol base.

Roller Blends

Roller ball bottles are a popular and convenient way to apply essential oils topically. Essential oils are pre-diluted in carrier oils and stored in roller ball bottles for easy application. Roller blends are generally used for targeted application to temples or specific areas of the body.

Are you a woman who appreciates the simplicity and effectiveness of roller blends? I love how they offer convenience for enjoying the benefits of essential oils with ease. With my collection of roller blends in hand, I create personalized, targeted applications.

One morning, I decided to prepare a blend that would uplift my mood and promote positivity throughout the day. I diluted my favorite citrus essential oils with a carrier oil and carefully filled a roller bottle. As I applied the blend to my temples, at the back of my ears, and on my wrists, I immediately felt a burst of freshness and energy. The invigorating scent lingered, serving as a constant reminder to embrace joy and positivity.

Later in the day, I felt the tension in my neck and shoulders, so I created a soothing roller blend to provide relief. In another roller bottle, I combined lavender and peppermint essential oils diluted in a carrier oil. With a gentle roll along the back of my neck and on my shoulders, I experienced the cooling sensation of peppermint and the calming properties of lavender. The blend worked wonders, helping me relax and unwind from the day's stress.

Although I often prefer to use citrus essential oils for a refreshing and uplifting effect, it's important to know that there are many other oils that can be used in roller blends. Essential oils like rose, valor, ylang-ylang, and frankincense each have their own unique benefits. For instance, frankincense can help with bruises and cold symptoms, while rose, valor, and ylang-ylang have calming properties.

Roller blends have become my go-to solution when I have a specific targeted need. I love how easy it is to apply my personalized blends wherever I go. Whether I need an energy boost, want to unwind, or support specific areas of my body, roller blends are an essential part of my self-care routine.

Rubs and Gels

Erica is a woman who loves incorporating essential oils into her daily self-care routine. She decided to create a soothing muscle rub using her favorite essential oils. She makes a comforting blend by adding a few droplets of peppermint, lavender, and eucalyptus to coconut oil.

After a long day of physical activity, she gently massages the rub onto her tired muscles. As the aromatic blend absorbs into her skin, she feels a wave of relaxation and relief wash over her. The soothing aroma and targeted application of the rub provide localized benefits, easing tension and promoting overall relaxation.

With her homemade essential oil rub, Erica finds solace in the power of natural remedies. Whether it's relieving muscle tension or promoting a sense of calm, these rubs and gels allow her to personalize her self-care and find moments of tranquility amidst the demands of her day.

Essential oils can be incorporated into gels or ointments to create topical applications. For example, you can create a soothing muscle rub by combining essential oils with a carrier substance like aloe vera gel or coconut oil. These rubs and gels can be applied to the skin for targeted relief.

These techniques allow for the targeted application of essential oils, providing localized benefits and overall relaxation. Each application technique has its benefits and considerations, and it's important to follow safety guidelines and dilution ratios for each method. Here's an example of an essential oil instruction label you can use on homemade products.

ESSENTIAL OILS INSTRUCTION LABEL

Up until now, we have explored the origins, extraction methods, quality considerations, and various application techniques for essential oils. Armed with this knowledge, we are now ready to look at the health aspects of using essential oils effectively.

4

THE ESSENTIAL OIL HEALTH GUIDE

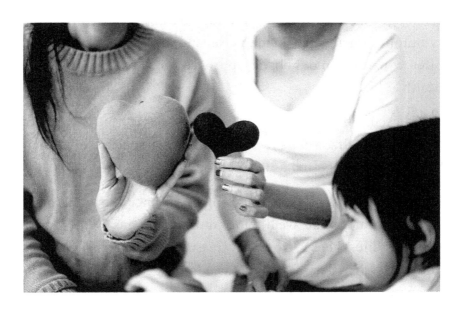

T his chapter is all about harnessing the power of essential oils for your health. Specifically, we're diving into how these oils can work wonders for your hormonal well-being. Think about more energy, better sleep, and improved intimacy. Trust me, it's a game-changer!

If you're wondering how essential oils can help with your hormonal health, you're in the right place. We've got some amazing information lined up to guide you through this exciting journey. Get ready to feel great—inside and out!

WOMEN'S HORMONE HEALTH AND ESSENTIAL OILS

Maintaining hormonal balance is key to women's overall well-being. Essential oils have been recognized for their potential to promote harmony within the body. Whether it's navigating the challenges of menstrual cycles, supporting fertility, or easing symptoms during perimenopause and beyond, essential oils offer a natural and holistic approach to women's hormonal health.

We'll discuss the best essential oils to support your hormonal health, providing valuable information on specific oils, their benefits, and suggested usage methods.

Essential oils can alleviate discomfort, balance hormones, and promote emotional well-being during various stages of a woman's life. These aromatic treasures hold transformative potential, from clary sage and lavender to geranium and frankincense.

It is important to remember that essential oils should be used mindfully and in conjunction with professional guidance. Always consult your healthcare provider before incorporating essential oils into your wellness routine, especially if you have specific health concerns or are on any medications.

Stress Management

Essential oils have gained recognition for their ability to provide support in stress management and promote emotional well-being. Their natural aromas and therapeutic properties can help ease stress, anxiety, and depression, boost feelings of relaxation, and improve sleep. Let's explore how essential oils can be effectively used for these purposes.

Using Essential Oils for Stress Relief

Certain essential oils possess calming and soothing properties that can help alleviate stress, reduce feelings of anxiety, and uplift moods. Many people use lavender oil for its calming scent, which is well-known for inducing relaxation. Other essential oils, such as bergamot, chamomile, and frankincense, are also known to improve mood and may reduce symptoms of depression and anxiety.

- Diffuse the oils: Add a few drops of bergamot essential oil to a diffuser and let the aroma fill the room, creating a calming atmosphere.
- Inhalation: Place a drop or two of lavender oil on a tissue or handkerchief and inhale deeply (*Practical Use of Essential Oils*, 2023). Alternatively, you can add a few drops to a personal inhaler for on-the-go stress relief.
- Bathing: Add a few drops of ylang ylang essential oil to your bathwater for a relaxing and aromatic experience.

Enhance Relaxation Using Essential Oils

Several essential oils have sedative properties that can help induce relaxation and promote a sense of tranquility. Oils such as clary sage, ylang-ylang, and vetiver are known for their ability to calm the mind and body.

- Create a calming massage blend: Combining aromatherapy during a massage can offer more significant and longer-lasting relief from fatigue, particularly mental fatigue, compared to massage alone. Mix a few drops of essential oil with a carrier oil, like sweet almond or jojoba oil, and gently massage it onto your skin.
- Pillow spray: Mix a few drops of essential oil with water in a spray bottle and spritz it onto your pillow before bedtime for a soothing aroma that promotes relaxation.

Using Essential Oils for Better Sleep

Essential oils have soothing and calming properties that can help improve sleep quality and alleviate insomnia. Lavender, chamomile, and sandalwood oils are popular choices for promoting restful sleep.

- Diffuse the oils in your bedroom: Use before going to bed to create a peaceful and sleep-inducing environment. Apply a diluted blend of essential oils to the soles of your feet or wrists before bedtime. Create a sleep-inducing linen spray by mixing essential oils with water and spraying it lightly on your bedsheets.

Energy Support

Hormonal changes can significantly impact a woman's energy levels, influencing her overall vitality and well-being (Neville, 2022). Understanding how hormones affect energy can provide you with valuable insights into managing fatigue and optimizing energy levels. Throughout your life, hormone levels fluctuate due to various factors, including your menstrual cycles, pregnancy, menopause, and hormonal imbalances. These hormonal shifts can directly impact your energy levels, often leading to changes in vitality and fatigue patterns (Charlotte, 2020).

- Menstrual cycle: The menstrual cycle involves hormonal fluctuations, particularly estrogen and progesterone. These hormones can influence energy levels in different phases of the cycle. Rising estrogen levels are associated with increased energy during the follicular phase (before ovulation). Conversely, during the luteal phase (after ovulation), progesterone levels rise, which can contribute to feelings of fatigue and decreased energy.
- Pregnancy: Pregnancy triggers significant hormonal changes, including increased progesterone and estrogen levels. While many women experience increased energy during the first trimester, fatigue often sets in during

the later stages due to hormonal shifts, increased
demands on the body, and changes in sleep patterns.
- Menopause: The transition into menopause is marked
by a decline in estrogen and progesterone production.
These hormonal changes can contribute to fatigue,
decreased energy levels, and disrupted sleep patterns in
women experiencing menopausal symptoms.

Hormonal imbalances, such as estrogen dominance or low
thyroid function, can also affect energy levels in women.
Estrogen dominance, where estrogen levels are relatively high
compared to progesterone, can lead to fatigue and mood
swings. Low thyroid function, known as hypothyroidism, can
cause fatigue, low energy, and a sluggish metabolism (Charlotte,
2020).

Managing energy levels during hormonal changes involves
adopting a holistic approach that addresses hormonal balance
and lifestyle factors. Doing this may include (*How Your
Hormones Affect Your Energy Levels - Thriva Health Hub*, 2023):

- Balancing hormones: Consulting with healthcare
professionals specializing in hormone optimization,
such as integrative or functional medicine practitioners,
can help identify and address hormonal imbalances
through personalized treatment plans.
- Managing stress: Chronic stress can impact your
hormone production and lead to fatigue. Implementing
stress management techniques like meditation, exercise,
and adequate rest can support your energy levels.

- Sleep hygiene: Prioritizing good sleep hygiene habits, such as establishing a regular sleep schedule, creating a relaxing bedtime routine, and optimizing your sleep environment, can help improve your energy levels.
- Balanced nutrition: Consuming a nutrient-dense diet that includes whole foods, healthy fats, and adequate protein can provide the necessary energy for your body. It is also necessary that you stay hydrated.

By understanding how hormonal changes influence energy levels and implementing strategies to support hormonal balance and overall well-being, women can optimize their energy levels and improve their quality of life.

Essential Oils for Mood and Coping

Several essential oils are known for their energizing properties. Here are some generally used essential oils for energy support (Frothingham, 2019):

- Peppermint: Known for its invigorating scent, peppermint oil can help increase alertness and mental clarity and boost energy levels.
- Sweet orange: The vibrant and citrusy aroma of sweet orange oil is often used to uplift mood, enhance focus, and promote a positive outlook.
- Rosemary: With its refreshing and herbaceous scent, rosemary oil is believed to enhance mental focus, improve cognitive performance, and combat mental fatigue.

- Lemon: The zesty and refreshing aroma of lemon oil can help promote energy, improve mood, and increase mental clarity.

Essential Oil Blends to Support Wellness

You can customize essential oil blends to provide specific energy support and promote well-being. Combining multiple essential oils creates synergistic effects that can enhance their individual properties. Some popular combinations for energy support include:

- Invigorating blend: Combining peppermint, lemon, and rosemary oils can create an uplifting and energizing blend to combat fatigue and increase alertness.
- Citrus blend: Blending sweet orange, lemon, and grapefruit oils can create a bright and refreshing aroma that promotes a positive mood and revitalizes the senses.
- Focus blend: Combining essential oils like peppermint, rosemary, and basil can enhance mental clarity and concentration and support sustained energy throughout the day.

Below is a list of essential oils to assist with energy, mood, and focus (Frothingham, 2019):

Essential oil	Benefits
Bergamot, cinnamon, ginger root, grapefruit, and pine	Enhances energy
Eucalyptus, thyme	Stimulates the brain, increases your mood, and boosts energy levels
Frankincense	Helps regulate the nervous system
French basil	Helps stimulate the adrenal glands
Juniper berry, lime, and wild orange	Improve your mood and inspire creativity
Lemon grass	Awakens your senses

Sleep Support

Hormone changes can significantly impact your sleep patterns, often leading to sleep quality and quantity disturbances. Understanding how hormones influence your sleep can provide valuable insights into managing sleep-related issues.

Throughout your life, hormonal fluctuations occur during various stages, including menstrual cycles, pregnancy, and menopause. These hormonal changes can influence sleep in the following ways:

- Menstrual cycle: Fluctuations in estrogen and progesterone levels during the menstrual cycle can affect sleep. Some women may experience difficulty falling asleep or staying asleep due to hormonal shifts. In particular, the premenstrual phase and the first few days of menstruation can be associated with disrupted sleep.
- Pregnancy: Hormonal changes during pregnancy, including increased levels of progesterone and

estrogen, can affect sleep patterns. Pregnant women may experience difficulty finding a comfortable sleeping position, frequent trips to the bathroom, and hormonal fluctuations that can disrupt sleep.

- Menopause: The transition into menopause involves a decline in estrogen and progesterone production. These hormonal changes can lead to various sleep disturbances, including insomnia, hot flashes, night sweats, and disrupted sleep patterns.

Hormonal imbalances, such as estrogen dominance or thyroid dysfunction, can also contribute to sleep disruptions. Estrogen dominance, where estrogen levels are relatively high compared to progesterone, can impact sleep quality and lead to insomnia. Low thyroid function (hypothyroidism) can cause symptoms such as fatigue, weight gain, and sleep disturbances.

Managing sleep disruptions during hormonal changes involves a comprehensive approach. In addition to stress management and boosting energy levels, getting better sleep will also address these problems.

Can Essential Oils Help You Sleep Better?

Did you know that one-third of adults in the United States struggle with getting enough sleep? It can be caused by difficulty falling or staying asleep (*CDC: Sleep and Sleep Disorders*, 2019). However, some essential oils have relaxing or sedative properties that may aid in promoting a better night's rest.

Many people choose to use essential oils for better sleep, and they have good reasons to do so. You can purchase these oils without a prescription; some research has shown promising results. Mahdavikian et al. (2020) did a study with 105 cardiac patients who had trouble sleeping. Those who breathed in peppermint and lavender oils slept better than those who only breathed in scented distilled water.

When inhaled, experts say that essential oils connect to the olfactory bulb in the nose. These oils trigger signals to the brain areas responsible for emotions and behavior, releasing neurotransmitters that can impact mood or behavior.

Three neurotransmitters affect our body and mind differently. Serotonin calms us and produces melatonin for sleep. Endorphins create euphoria and drowsiness, while noradrenaline stimulates us.

Which Oil Blends to Use?

Here are some of the most popular essential oil blends for sleep:

- Lavender: Lavender is often called the king of essential oils and is a crucial addition to any list. It has been proven to aid in sleep by reducing symptoms of insomnia and promoting slow-wave sleep, which is vital for feeling rested upon waking up in the morning.
- Chamomile: Chamomile is a well-known tea for promoting sleep, and it's believed that inhaling the scent of chamomile essential oil may have similar benefits. This oil is also thought to alleviate minor aches and pains as well as combat sleep deprivation.
- Clary sage: If you struggle with anxious thoughts that prevent you from sleeping, consider using clary sage.

This natural remedy is thought to have a calming effect on the mind and can reduce anxiety by lowering cortisol levels, which is the body's primary stress hormone. Clary sage may also function as a natural antidepressant due to its stress-reducing properties.

- Valerian: Valerian root is known for its soothing properties and is called a natural alternative to valium. Valerian essential oils may potentially aid in treating insomnia by helping you fall asleep faster.
- Vanilla: Vanilla's aroma is strong and recognizable, evoking many happy memories. As a result, it's one of the most generally used essential oils for promoting sleep and is believed to decrease stress and blood pressure, leading to a peaceful and restful night's rest.

Cravings and Weight Challenges

For Cravings

Cravings can sometimes feel overpowering, but fear not! Let's talk about why they happen and how essential oils can help manage them. Cravings often have a mischievous combination of psychological, hormonal, and physiological triggers that can throw us off track (Harvard School of Public Health, n.d.).

Fear not, aromatic adventurer! Essential oils are here to save the day, infusing our lives with a dash of whimsy and helping us conquer those cravings. Picture this: as you inhale the tantalizing scents of essential oils, your cravings retreat, almost as if they're being chased away by a troupe of mischievous aroma fairies.

In the realm of aromatherapy, where enchantment and fragrance reign supreme, peppermint and grapefruit oils reveal the secrets of essential oils for cravings. These potent elixirs and others like clove, cinnamon, and bergamot hold remarkable powers to support our cravings and lead us toward balance and wellness.

Almost like a magic potion, essential oils captivate our senses and cast a spell of positivity upon us, pulling our attention away from those pesky cravings like our favorite chocolate chip cookies, ice cream, or a bag of chips. Imagine grapefruit and orange oils stepping onto the stage, their zesty and uplifting aromas orchestrating a symphony of joy within us, effectively dampening the desire to reach for that tempting bag of chips (Barton, 2018).

Certain essential oils have the ability to harmonize our hormones, a crucial piece of the cravings puzzle. Behold the enchanting clary sage and lavender oils! With a swish of their aromatic wands, they work their magic to regulate hormones, whisking away stress and bestowing upon us a calm and serene state of mind (Barton, 2018).

There's more to this whimsical tale! Essential oils can even lend a hand in quelling our ravenous appetites. Enter peppermint oil, the mischievous trickster! Inhale its invigorating scent, and it might just give your cravings a playful poke. This delightful aroma provides a refreshing and satisfying sensation, giving you the upper hand in your quest to resist that decadent chocolate cake (Barton, 2018).

Welcome, fellow aroma enthusiasts! Discover the world of essential oils and unlock their captivating fragrances and practical benefits. Enrich your surroundings by infusing them with these delightful scents, or apply the oils creatively to enhance your experiences. These oils will accompany you on your journey towards healthier choices and a balanced lifestyle, bringing joy and inspiration to your everyday routines.

Remember, cravings may knock on your door, but with essential oils as your allies, you can greet them with a mischievous grin and bid them adieu. Let the fragrant magic guide you towards a life filled with vitality and flavor, where cravings become mere whispers in the wind.

Weight Challenges

Our bodies can sometimes present us with unique challenges when it comes to our weight. Let's explore the different aspects of weight management and discover how both oils can assist us in achieving our desired goals.

Weight Gain

Gaining weight can be a goal for some individuals who wish to build muscle mass or increase their overall body weight. Certain foods can aid in healthy weight gain (Khare, 2018). While oils are not a direct source of weight gain, you can use them with a well-balanced diet to support the process.

For example, healthy oils like olive, coconut, and avocado oils are rich in healthy fats and calories. You can incorporate these oils into meals to increase calorie intake and provide nourishment. When used in moderation and as part of a balanced diet, they can help individuals meet their weight gain goals (Khare, 2018).

Weight Loss

On the other hand, weight loss is a common goal for many of us seeking a healthier body composition. Essential oils can be a valuable addition to a weight loss journey by supporting various aspects of the process.

Certain essential oils have properties that can aid in weight loss efforts. For example, grapefruit essential oil is believed to have metabolism-boosting properties, which may help increase calorie burning and support weight loss. Lemon essential oil is known for its detoxifying effects, helping to cleanse the body and promote overall wellness. Peppermint essential oil can provide a refreshing and energizing sensation, potentially reducing cravings and assisting in portion control (Sullivan, 2023; Purdie, 2016).

Essential oils can be incorporated into a weight loss routine through aromatherapy, topical application, or ingestion, depending on the specific oil and its recommended usage. You should use essential oils safely and follow proper guidelines. It is important to still regularly exercise and eat healthy.

Weight management is a journey that requires a holistic approach. While essential oils can be a helpful addition to your routine, it's necessary to prioritize a well-balanced diet, regular physical activity, and overall lifestyle habits that support your goals. With the right mindset, dedication, and the assistance of essential oils, you can embark on a rewarding path toward achieving and maintaining a healthy weight.

Libido and Intimacy

Imagine a world where your hormonal changes no longer control your desires. Let's explore the fascinating connection between hormones and libido in women and discover simple ways to reignite your passion. Picture the incredible potential of essential oils as we introduce five irresistible blends that can boost your sexual drive.

- Ylang-ylang and jasmine blend: Close your eyes and breathe in the alluring scents of ylang-ylang and jasmine. They create a captivating blend that stirs desire and sets the mood.
- Rose and sandalwood blend: Imagine the delicate fragrance of roses mingling with sandalwood's warm and comforting scent. This enchanting blend can evoke feelings of romance and ignite your inner fire.
- Patchouli and neroli blend: Picture the earthy notes of patchouli harmonizing with the uplifting essence of neroli. This soothing blend can create a sensual atmosphere and promote relaxation.
- Ginger and cardamom blend: Feel the refreshing kick of ginger combined with the spicy allure of cardamom. This blend adds a touch of excitement and can awaken your senses.
- Clary sage and bergamot blend: Imagine the calming properties of clary sage blending with the uplifting

qualities of bergamot. This harmonious blend can restore balance and create a sense of well-being.

Exploring the potential benefits of essential oils for libido and intimacy can be an exciting journey. It is important to seek professional medical advice for any concerns or health conditions. By using care and consideration, you can make informed choices and find the best essential oils for your intimate experiences.

Perimenopause and Menopause

As women, we undergo significant hormonal changes during perimenopause and menopause that can impact our overall well-being. Menopause signifies the end of a woman's reproductive years, whereas perimenopause is the time leading up to it. Let's delve into these hormonal shifts and explore how essential oils can provide support during this transformative time.

During perimenopause, Suzie, a 40-year-old female, experienced fluctuating hormone levels. These changes resulted in hot flashes, irregular menstrual cycles, night sweats, and unbearable mood swings.

While Suzie understood that essential oils couldn't directly address hormonal imbalances, she was hopeful that they might offer some relief for the symptoms she was experiencing. She discovered that some essential oils possess properties that promote relaxation, alleviate stress, improve sleep quality, and enhance overall well-being, which could indirectly support me during this transitional phase.

Suzie wondered, *"Can essential oils help me?"* She realized that they were not a replacement for medical treatment, but they could complement her existing strategies for managing menopausal symptoms. She learned that a blend of lavender and clary sage oils might help balance her hormones and promote relaxation and emotional well-being. She tried a combination of geranium and rose oils to create a comforting and uplifting atmosphere, potentially assisting with hormone balancing. Suzie also found that a blend of peppermint and lemon oils, with their cooling and mood-enhancing properties, could potentially provide relief during times of discomfort, particularly when managing hot flashes.

It was important for her to remember that essential oils should be used with caution and in appropriate dilutions. She understood that essential oils were just one part of a holistic approach to managing perimenopause and menopause. Suzie embraced a balanced diet, engaged in regular exercise, practiced stress management techniques, and sought medical advice when necessary. By incorporating essential oils into her overall wellness journey during this transformative phase, she experienced their potential benefits and found comfort and support along the way.

Blends to Try

While individual preferences may vary, here are a few essential oil blends that have been suggested for managing menopausal symptoms:

- Lavender and clary sage blend: Clary sage may aid in balancing hormones, while lavender oil is well-known for its relaxing effects. Combining these oils in a blend could potentially promote relaxation and emotional well-being.
- Geranium and rose blend: Geranium oil has been associated with hormone-balancing effects, and rose oil is often used for its soothing aroma. Blending these oils may create a comforting and uplifting atmosphere.
- Peppermint and lemon blend: Peppermint oil offers a cooling sensation and may assist with managing hot flashes, while lemon oil is believed to have mood-enhancing properties. This invigorating blend may help provide relief during times of discomfort.

SPA RECIPES AT HOME

Imagine treating yourself to a blissful spa day in the comfort of your own home. As a woman, mother, or grandmother you deserve a well-deserved break and some relaxation. Let's have a look at some wonderful spa recipes that use essential oils to help you relax and rejuvenate.

- Relaxing bath soak: Start your spa day by indulging in a luxurious bath soak. Add one cup of Epsom salt, one tablespoon of carrier oil, and ten drops of lavender essential oil to a warm bath. The soothing scent of lavender will allow you to unwind.
- Nourishing facial steam: Do a facial steam to open up your pores and rejuvenate your skin. Boil a pot of water

and pour it into a heatproof bowl. Add three to five droplets of your favorite essential oil, such as geranium or rose, known for their nourishing and balancing properties. Place a towel over your head, lean over the bowl, and let the steam envelop your face for 5–10 minutes.

- Relaxation massage oil: Treat yourself to a soothing self-massage with homemade massage oil. In a small bottle, combine 1/4 cup of carrier oil (such as coconut or grapeseed oil) with 10 droplets of your preferred essential oil blend. For relaxation, consider a blend of lavender, chamomile, and bergamot. Gently massage the oil into your skin, focusing on areas of tension and stress.

- Calming room diffuser blend: Create a serene atmosphere in your spa space by diffusing a calming essential oil blend. In a diffuser, add water and five to eight droplets of essential oils like lavender, ylang-ylang, and frankincense. The gentle and soothing aroma will help create a tranquil ambiance, promoting a sense of peace and relaxation.

- Refreshing body scrub: Treat your skin to a revitalizing body scrub. In a bowl, combine half a cup of sea salt or sugar with a quarter cup of carrier oil (such as jojoba or almond). Add 10 droplets of your favorite essential oil, such as grapefruit or peppermint, known for its invigorating and uplifting qualities. Gently massage the scrub onto damp skin in circular motions, then rinse off for soft and smooth skin.

Relaxation Massage Oil

Ingredients

- A quarter cup of almond oil
- 20 drops of lavender essential oil
- Six drops of cedarwood oil
- 10 drops of sweet orange oil

Directions

1. In a small bottle or container, pour a quarter cup of almond oil.
2. Add 20 drops of lavender essential oil to the almond oil.
3. Then, add six drops of cedarwood essential oil.
4. At last, add 10 drops of sweet orange essential oil to the combination.
5. Secure the bottle with a lid and shake well to thoroughly blend the oils.

When you're ready to unwind and de-stress, pour a small amount of the oil into your palms, warm it between your hands, and gently massage it onto your body. Breathe in the soothing aromas of lavender, cedarwood, and sweet orange as you relax and enjoy the calming effects of this massage oil (Carter, 2022).

PERSONAL SKIN AND HAIR CARE RECIPES

Being a busy woman or mother, it's important to prioritize self-care, including taking care of your skin and hair. Essential oils can be a wonderful addition to your beauty routine, providing natural benefits and a touch of luxury. Let's explore some personal skin and hair care recipes using essential oils that will benefit you:

Toning Face Mask with Essential Oils

Ingredients

- Three tablespoons of pure aloe gel (alcohol-free) (carrier oil)
- Three tablespoons of raw, unfiltered honey
- Five drops of cucumber seed oil
- One drop of cedarwood oil
- Four drops of red mandarin oil

Note: The recipe makes a larger quantity, but it provides a subtle hint of cedarwood.

Directions

1. Before using the face mask, perform a patch test on the back of your hand or the bottom of your foot to ensure it won't cause irritation.
2. Carefully avoid the eye area when applying and removing the mask (avoid eyelids and areas below the eyebrows; they may appear shiny due to lighting).

3. In a bowl, thoroughly mix all the ingredients together.

4. Apply the mixture evenly to your skin, covering your face.

5. Relax for approximately ten to fifteen minutes while allowing the mask to dry on your skin.

6. To remove the mask, use a hot washcloth and gently wipe it off.

With the refreshing aromas of cucumber seed, cedarwood, and red mandarin essential oils, enjoy the toning benefits of this face mask (Homemade Cucumber Mandarin Face Mask with Essential Oils, 2016).

Nourishing Face Serum

Ingredients

- Two tablespoons of jojoba oil
- Five drops of rosehip seed oil
- Three drops of frankincense oil
- Two drops of lavender oil

Directions

In a small bottle or container, combine the jojoba oil and rosehip seed oil. Add the lavender and frankincense oils. Mix well. Apply a few droplets of this nourishing serum to your clean face in the morning and evening. The blend of oils will hydrate your skin and promote a youthful complexion.

Soothing Body Scrub

Ingredients

- Half a cup of sugar (white or brown)
- Two tablespoons of coconut oil (carrier)
- Five drops of lavender essential oil
- Three drops of chamomile essential oil

Directions

In a bowl, combine the sugar and coconut oil until they form a scrub-like consistency. Blend the chamomile and lavender oils. Gently massage the scrub into your damp skin in small circles, paying special attention to dry or rough areas (Axe, 2022). Rinse off with warm water, and enjoy the calming and soothing effects of this aromatic body scrub.

Nourishing Facial Oil

Ingredients

- Two tablespoons of jojoba oil (carrier)
- Four drops of lavender oil
- Two drops of frankincense oil
- Two drops of geranium oil

Directions

Blend jojoba oil with lavender, then frankincense, and finally geranium essential oils in a small container. After cleansing your face, apply a few droplets of this nourishing facial oil to your skin. Gently massage it using small upward circle movements. Allow the oil to absorb before applying any additional products. This blend will provide hydration, promote a healthy complexion, and leave your skin feeling nourished.

Soothing Body Lotion

Ingredients

- Half a cup of shea butter
- Two tablespoons of coconut oil (carrier)
- Ten drops of chamomile oil
- Five drops of rose oil

Directions

In a bowl that won't melt, heat the shea butter and coconut oil together. Once melted, let it cool for a few minutes. Add the chamomile and rose essential oils to the mixture and stir well. Place the bowl in the refrigerator for about 10–15 minutes to allow the mixture to solidify slightly. Remove the mixture from the refrigerator and whip it using an electric mixer until it becomes creamy and fluffy. Transfer the soothing body lotion to a clean jar or container. Apply this lotion all over your body after bathing or whenever your skin needs hydration and soothing. The chamomile and rose essential oils will help calm and nourish your skin, leaving it soft and supple.

Revitalizing Hair Mask

Ingredients

- Two tablespoons of coconut oil
- One tablespoon of honey
- Five droplets of peppermint oil
- Three droplets of rosemary oil

Directions

In a bowl, melt the honey and coconut oil together. Add the peppermint and rosemary essential oils and mix thoroughly. Apply the mask to wet hair, paying special attention to the ends and any broken areas. Leave it on for 20–30 minutes, then rinse it out and shampoo as usual. This rejuvenating mask will nourish your hair, leaving it soft, shiny, and revitalized.

Hair Shampoo Recipe

Ingredients

- Ten droplets of lavender essential oil
- Five droplets of rosemary oil
- Five droplets of peppermint oil
- 11 cups of liquid castile soap
- 1/4 cup of coconut milk
- One tablespoon of almond oil (carrier)

Directions

1. Combine the liquid castile soap, canned coconut milk, and almond oil in a bowl or jar.
2. Add the lavender, rosemary, and peppermint essential oils to the mixture.
3. Stir well to ensure all the ingredients are thoroughly blended.
4. Transfer the shampoo mixture to a bottle or container with a flip-top or pump dispenser for easy use.
5. Gently shake the bottle prior to each use to mix the ingredients.

To use the shampoo, wet your hair thoroughly and then apply a small amount of the homemade shampoo to your scalp. Massage gently to create a lather, and work the shampoo through your hair. Rinse well with water. Apply a conditioner if you like to.

This homemade shampoo recipe combines the cleansing properties of castile soap with the moisturizing effects of coconut milk and almond oil. The lavender, rosemary, and peppermint essential oils not only add a pleasant aroma but may also provide benefits such as promoting hair growth, reducing scalp irritation, and improving overall hair health (Nelson, 2013).

Incorporating these personal skin and hair care recipes into your routine will not only provide nourishment and rejuvenation but also allow you to indulge in some well-deserved self-care moments amidst your busy schedule.

As we move forward to the next chapter, I invite you to explore a specific application of essential oils: their use by men. In the fifth chapter, "Beyond After-Shave Cologne - Oils for Men," we explore essential oils that focus on men's health and wellness. Learn how these oils can improve vitality and emotional well-being and address specific concerns unique to men. However, before you move on to the next chapter, use this handy template to list your favorite essential oils.

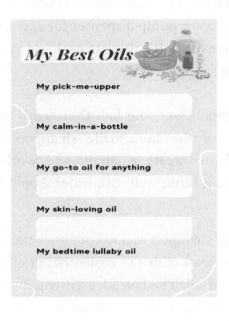

I WOULD LOVE TO HEAR FROM YOU!

Your feedback and support have played an instrumental role in extending the reach of my book, "Aromatherapy for Self Care," to a diverse audience of women, mothers, grandmothers, and beyond.

I would be deeply appreciative if you could spare a moment to share your insights and impressions about my book.

I invite you to kindly consider leaving a review on Amazon once it becomes available. Thank you wholeheartedly for your unwavering support, which continues to inspire and drive my passion for aromatherapy and self-care.

Scan the QR code below

5

BEYOND AFTERSHAVE—OILS FOR MEN

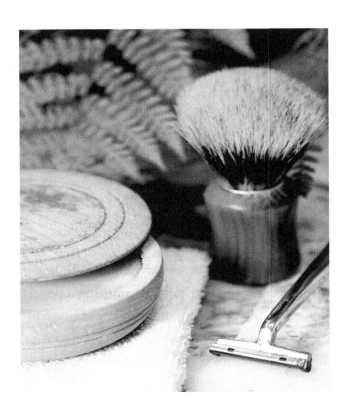

Wouldn't it be great if the men in our lives could also benefit from this book? I've added this chapter specifically with them in mind. Whether you give it to them to read on their own or share the tips you've found here with them in conversation, I hope they will also greatly benefit from the power of essential oils.

Aromatherapy, often associated with women, also holds immense benefits for men. From natural mood enhancement to improved sleep quality, heightened focus, and overall health benefits, essential oils offer a holistic approach to supporting men's well-being.

- Natural mood booster: Aromatherapy can uplift mood and promote emotional balance in men. Essential oils such as cedarwood, vetiver, and sandalwood have grounding and soothing properties that can help relieve stress, anxiety, and tension. By incorporating these oils into their daily routine, men can experience a natural mood boost and a greater sense of calm.
- Quality of sleep: Getting a good night's sleep is crucial for overall health and well-being. Aromatherapy can play a significant role in improving sleep quality for men. Essential oils like lavender, chamomile, and clary sage are relaxing and soothing, promoting a peaceful environment and preparing the mind and body for restful sleep. Discover how these oils can create a soothing bedtime ritual and enhance the quality of your sleep.

- Improved focus: In a world filled with distractions, maintaining focus and mental clarity can be challenging. Aromatherapy offers a natural solution to improve concentration and enhance cognitive performance. Essential oils like rosemary, peppermint, and lemon have invigorating and stimulating properties that help sharpen focus, boost productivity, and increase mental alertness. Explore the benefits of these oils and learn how to incorporate them into your daily routine.
- Overall health benefits: Aromatherapy goes beyond mood and sleep. Essential oils can contribute to men's overall health and well-being. Certain oils, such as tea tree, eucalyptus, and frankincense, possess antimicrobial and immune-boosting properties. Discover how these oils can support respiratory health, promote healthy skin, and contribute to a more robust immune system.

ESSENTIAL OILS FOR MEN

Hey, guys! If you're looking to explore the wonderful world of essential oils, you might be wondering which ones are suitable for men. Look no further, and let's discover the essential oils that can best complement and enhance men's overall wellness.

Imagine running through a lush forest, surrounded by towering trees and the earthy scent of nature. Or picture yourself in a vibrant spice market, where the air is filled with the warm and enticing aroma of exotic spices. These sensory experiences can be captured and enjoyed through the use of essential oils. Men, in particular, can benefit from the unique qualities of certain essential oils that align with their preferences and needs. Let's explore some must-have categories of essential oils for men: woods, earthy, spicy, minty, and citrus.

Woody Essential Oils

Think of the rugged and robust scents that evoke images of strength and masculinity. Cedarwood, sandalwood, and vetiver are perfect examples. These oils not only have an appealing woody fragrance but also provide a calming and grounding effect, making them ideal for promoting a sense of stability and inner strength (*Feel Handsome, Smell Awesome: 7 Essential Oils for Men*, 2019).

Earthy Essential Oils

These oils bring forth the essence of the great outdoors. Imagine walking through a serene forest after a rainstorm, where the damp soil and green foliage combine to create a soothing ambiance. Essential oils like patchouli, frankincense, and myrrh can recreate that experience, helping men feel connected to nature and fostering a sense of balance and tranquility.

Spicy Essential Oils

For those who seek a more intense and passionate aroma, spicy essential oils are the way to go. Picture yourself in a bustling kitchen, where the air is filled with the invigorating scents of black pepper, ginger, and cinnamon. These oils have a warm and stimulating effect, adding a dash of excitement and energy to your daily routine.

Minty Essential Oils

If you crave a fresh and invigorating scent, minty essential oils will be your go-to. Imagine the crisp, cool sensation you get from chewing on a refreshing mint leaf. Essential oils like peppermint, spearmint, and wintergreen can provide that same burst of freshness, awakening your senses and revitalizing your mind and body.

Citrus Essential Oils

Citrus essential oils offer a bright and uplifting fragrance. Imagine yourself on a sunny morning, sipping freshly squeezed orange juice as the citrusy aroma envelops you. Essential oils such as lemon, orange, and grapefruit have a zesty and invigorating effect, promoting positivity and a sense of optimism.

INCORPORATING ESSENTIAL OILS INTO YOUR ROUTINE

Here are some essential oil blends you can use in different aspects of your daily routine:

For the office

- Blend one: Blend three droplets of cedarwood, three droplets of bergamot, and two droplets of Frankincense essential oil together. This blend promotes focus, productivity, and a calm atmosphere.

- Blend two: To create a refreshing blend that may enhance mental clarity and alertness, mix four droplets of peppermint, two droplets of rosemary, and two droplets of lemon essential oil.

Nightlife

- Blend one: Craft an alluring combination by combining three droplets of sandalwood, two droplets of patchouli, and two droplets of ylang-ylang essential oil. This blend is alluring and promotes confidence.
- Blend two: Blend three droplets of vetiver, two droplets of black pepper, and two droplets of bergamot essential oil. This blend offers a subtle, masculine scent and energizes the senses.

Outdoor

- Blend one: Combine three droplets of eucalyptus, three drops of tea tree, and two droplets of peppermint essential oil. This mixture has a pleasant scent and can help repel pests.
- Blend two: Blend three droplets of lemongrass, two droplets of cedarwood, and two droplets of lavender essential oil. This combination is soothing and energizing.

Lemon cedar

- Combine four droplets of lemon and three droplets of cedarwood essential oil. This blend has a fresh, citrusy aroma with grounding notes of cedar.

Floral mint

- Mix three droplets of lavender, two droplets of peppermint, and two droplets of clary sage essential oil. This blend incorporates a soothing floral scent with a cool minty freshness.

Fresh and clean

- Blend one: Combine four droplets of grapefruit, two drops of lemon, and two droplets of rosemary essential oil. This blend has a refreshing citrus scent.
- Blend two: Mix three droplets of lemongrass, two droplets of bergamot, and two droplets of eucalyptus essential oil. This blend offers a clean and uplifting aroma.

Citrus

- Combine equal parts of lemon, orange, and grapefruit essential oils. This blend provides an energizing and refreshing citrusy scent.

Earthy blends

- Blend one: Mix three droplets of patchouli, two droplets of vetiver, and two droplets of bergamot essential oil. The blend has a grounding and earthy aroma.
- Blend two: Mix two droplets of cedarwood, three droplets of frankincense, and two droplets of sandalwood essential oil. The blend promotes relaxation and tranquility.

Woodsy blends

- Blend one: Mix three droplets of cypress, two droplets of cedarwood, and two droplets of juniper berry essential oil. This blend has a forest-like aroma that evokes a sense of grounding.
- Blend two: Combine three droplets of pine, two droplets of sandalwood, and two droplets of bergamot essential oil. The blend offers a woodsy and uplifting scent.

Here are some ideas for how you can use essential oils in your daily life:

- Personal fragrance: Create your own signature scent by blending essential oils with carrier oils, such as jojoba or almond oil. Simply add a few drops of your preferred oil, such as cedarwood, sandalwood, or vetiver, to a carrier oil of your choice. For an attractive scent, rub the blend on your wrists, throat, or behind your ears.

- Diffusing: Invest in an essential oil diffuser to fill your living space with the enchanting aroma of woody oils. Add a few drops of your favorite woody or citrus oil to the diffuser along with water, and let the diffuser disperse the scent throughout the room. This is a great way to create a calming and grounding atmosphere, especially after a long day.
- Bath soak: After a hectic day, treat yourself to a relaxing bath infused with minty essential oils. Immerse yourself in a soothing and aromatic experience by adding a few drops of your preferred oil to your bathwater. The warm water will help release the aroma, enveloping you in a tranquil ambiance while rejuvenating your mind and body.
- Massage: Arrange a soothing massage session and request the use of woody essential oils as part of the massage oil blend. The calming and grounding properties of woody oils can enhance the massage experience, promoting relaxation and relieving tension in your muscles.
- Personal care products: Enhance your grooming routine by adding earthy essential oils to your personal care products. You can mix a few drops of spicy oil with your shampoo, body wash, or facial cleanser for a refreshing and grounding experience. The natural fragrances of these oils will invigorate your senses and provide a touch of luxury to your self-care routine.

- DIY grooming products: Get creative and incorporate essential oils into your grooming routine. You can add a few drops of cedarwood or sandalwood oil to your shaving cream or aftershave for a delightful fragrance that lingers. You could also infuse your beard oil or beard balm with vetiver essential oil for a unique and masculine scent.
- DIY home care products: Get creative and make your own home care products infused with earthy essential oils. You can add a few drops of oils like patchouli or frankincense to homemade cleaning solutions or create your own room sprays by mixing earthy oils with water in a spray bottle. This way, you can enjoy the benefits of these oils while keeping your living environment fresh and naturally scented.

Whether you choose to wear them as a personal fragrance, enjoy them through diffusion, indulge in a luxurious bath, incorporate them into your grooming routine, or explore other creative methods, woody essential oils can bring a touch of nature and masculinity to your daily life.

ESSENTIAL OILS IN YOUR SKINCARE ROUTINE

Essential oils can help with your skincare for many reasons, such as soothing irritation, promoting healthy skin, and providing a refreshing scent. Here are some essential oil blends that are appropriate for men to use:

- Refreshing aftershave blend: Combine two droplets of cedarwood, two droplets of lavender, and two droplets of tea tree essential oil with one tablespoon of carrier oil, such as jojoba or almond.
- Beard oil blend: Blend three droplets of sandalwood, two droplets of bergamot, and two droplets of cedarwood essential oil with 1 ounce of carrier oil, such as argan or jojoba. This blend can promote a healthy-looking beard and moisturize the skin underneath.
- Acne-fighting blend: Combine two droplets of tea tree, two droplets of lavender, and two droplets of frankincense essential oil with one tablespoon of aloe vera gel or a non-comedogenic carrier oil. This blend can help combat acne, reduce inflammation, and promote clearer skin.
- Skin-soothing blend: Mix three droplets of chamomile, two droplets of helichrysum, and two droplets of lavender essential oil with one tablespoon of aloe vera gel or carrier oil. This blend is soothing and can help alleviate skin irritation or redness.
- Anti-aging blend: Combine two droplets of frankincense, two droplets of geranium, and two droplets of patchouli essential oil with one tablespoon of a carrier oil that is rich in antioxidants, such as rosehip seed or pomegranate seed oil.
- Energizing facial mist: Mix five droplets of peppermint, three droplets of eucalyptus, and two droplets of lemon essential oil with two ounces of distilled water. Shake well and use it as a refreshing facial mist to invigorate the skin and awaken the senses.

- Calming nighttime blend: Combine three droplets of lavender, two droplets of vetiver, and two droplets of Roman chamomile essential oil with one tablespoon of carrier oil. The blend promotes relaxation. Apply it before bedtime to support peaceful sleep and rejuvenate your skin.

ESSENTIAL OIL RECIPES FOR MEN

Here are some recipes using essential oils that can address specific concerns for men:

- Headache relief: You can blend two droplets of peppermint, two droplets of lavender, and two droplets of eucalyptus essential oil. Mix the blend with one tablespoon of a carrier oil, like coconut or almond oil, to make it less strong. Apply a small amount to the temples and back of the neck to relieve headaches.
- Stress relief: You can combine two droplets of vetiver, two droplets of frankincense, and three droplets of bergamot essential oil. Weaken (dilute) the blend with one tablespoon of carrier oil. Apply topically or diffuse.
- Focus or memory: You can blend three droplets of rosemary, two droplets of peppermint, and two droplets of lemon essential oil. Diffuse the blend while studying, working, or needing mental clarity. You can also create a personal inhaler by adding the blend to a cotton wick or a nasal inhaler.
- Hair loss: You can mix three droplets of cedarwood, two droplets of rosemary, and two droplets of lavender

essential oil. Weaken the blend with one tablespoon of carrier oil. Massage a small amount into the scalp to stimulate hair growth and improve the condition of the scalp.

- Shaving oils: You can blend two droplets of sandalwood, two droplets of tea tree, and two droplets of cedarwood essential oil. Dilute the blend in one tablespoon of carrier oil. Apply a small amount to the face before shaving to moisturize the skin, reduce irritation, and provide a smooth shave.
- Sore muscles: You can combine three droplets of peppermint, two droplets of eucalyptus, and two droplets of lavender essential oil. Weaken the blend with one tablespoon of carrier oil. Massage the blend into the affected areas to soothe sore muscles and reduce inflammation.

Now that we've gone over essential oils specifically tailored to men, let's help out the mothers and focus on essential oils for children, exploring different blends suitable for various age groups. We will discuss essential oil safety guidelines for kids and recommend age-appropriate blends. Whether you have infants, toddlers, or older children, this chapter will help you navigate the world of essential oils and make informed choices for your little ones' well-being. Stay tuned to discover how essential oils can support your children's health and promote a nurturing environment for their growth and development.

6

THE MOTHER'S GUIDE TO ESSENTIAL OILS—FINDING THE PERFECT BLEND FOR YOUR CHILD'S AGE

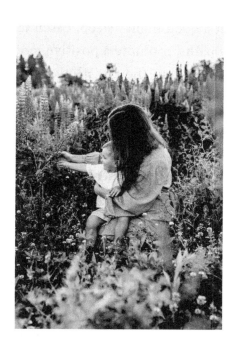

A s a mother, you're well aware that it's not an easy job. You have to deal with stress, fatigue, mood swings, and a lack of sleep. Essential oils can be of great help in managing these challenges, providing a natural and holistic solution. Imagine coming home after a long day at work and finding chaos at home. But you remember that you have a bottle of lavender essential oil in your handbag. You diffuse it in the living room, and the soothing scent helps to lower your stress levels and calm your mind. You're able to tackle your chores with renewed energy and a sense of peace. Essential oils can also help you with sleep issues (Axe, 2022). A few drops of chamomile essential oil on your pillow can help you relax and get a good night's sleep. Essential oils can soothe minor aches and pains, promote a positive mood, and help you stay energized throughout the day. However, it's important to always use them safely and seek the guidance of a qualified healthcare practitioner.

Essential oils are the secret weapon every mother needs in her arsenal. With the power of essential oils, you can conquer almost anything that comes your way and do it all with a smile on your face!

ARE ESSENTIAL OILS SAFE FOR PREGNANCY?

Pregnancy is a special time for women, and the use of essential oils should be approached with caution to ensure the safety of both the mother and the developing baby. Let's explore the topic further:

When it comes to using essential oils during pregnancy, it is important to consider their safety. While some essential oils can provide benefits, others may pose risks. It is always best to consult with a healthcare professional for guidance on the safe use of oils during pregnancy.

To use essential oils safely during pregnancy, consider the following guidelines:

- Manage your morning sickness: Certain essential oils can help alleviate symptoms of morning sickness. However, it is crucial to choose oils that are considered safe during pregnancy.
- Treat your bump to a bath soak: Enjoying a relaxing bath with certain essential oils can provide relief during pregnancy.
- Uplift and calm yourself during labor: Essential oils can create a soothing atmosphere during labor.
- Help with postpartum: Essential oils can also be beneficial during the postpartum period.

There are some essential oils that you shouldn't use when you're pregnant because they could be dangerous. It is recommended to steer clear of these oils to ensure the well-being of both yourself and your baby. A list of oils to avoid will be provided as we continue discussing oil safety.

Some essential oils are generally considered safe for use during pregnancy and breastfeeding. The following essential oil options may be considered after the first trimester of your pregnancy: lavender, peppermint, lemon, geranium, chamomile, rose, ginger, cardamom, argon, patchouli, and frankincense.

It is always best to consult with a healthcare professional, such as a midwife or obstetrician, before using essential oils during pregnancy.

ESSENTIAL OILS AND NEW MOMS

As a new mom, you'll go through a transformative journey both during pregnancy and after childbirth. Essential oils can provide support and comfort during this precious time. Let's look at how new moms can use essential oils:

- Oils to avoid for newborn babies: When it comes to using essential oils around newborn babies, it is important to exercise caution. Some essential oils may be too strong or potentially harmful for their delicate systems. It is generally recommended to avoid using essential oils directly on or around newborn babies.
- Oils to avoid during pregnancy and breastfeeding: There are some essential oils that you shouldn't use while you're pregnant or breastfeeding because they could cause harm to the baby or the mother. It is important to be cautious when using essential oils during pregnancy and while breastfeeding, as exceeding the recommended dosage can pose a risk of toxicity. Essential oils, like sage, basil, aniseed, wormwood, mugwort, tarragon, rue, oak moss, birch, hyssop, camphor, parsley, pennyroyal, tansy, thuja, and

wintergreen, should be avoided when you are pregnant
or breastfeeding (Dessinger, 2016).

- How to diffuse essential oils for newborns: Diffusing
  essential oils can create a pleasant atmosphere for both
  the newborn and the mother. Here are some secure
  ways to use essential oils for newborns:
- Sleep time: Diffusing calming essential oils like
  lavender or chamomile in the nursery before bedtime
  can help create a soothing environment for better sleep.
- Awake time: During awake and playtime, uplifting
  essential oils such as citrus or peppermint can provide a
  refreshing and energizing ambiance.
- Boosting their immune system: Essential oils that help
  the immune system, like tea tree or lemon, can be
  diffused to promote a healthy environment.
- Breathing ease: For respiratory support, diffusing
  gentle essential oils like eucalyptus or frankincense can
  help promote easy breathing.
- Diluting essential oils for newborns: When using
  essential oils for newborns, it is important to dilute
  them properly. Dilution helps make sure that the
  application is safe and gentle (McDermott, 2017). Dilute
  essential oils in a carrier oil, such as fractionated
  coconut oil or jojoba oil, before using them on your
  skin (Axe, 2022).
- Roller bottle blends: Roller bottle blends are a
  convenient way to apply diluted essential oils to specific
  areas. Here are a few roller bottle blends suitable for
  new moms:

- Calming and sleep: A blend of Roman chamomile, lavender, and vetiver diluted in a carrier oil can help promote relaxation and better sleep.
- Tummy discomfort: A blend of ginger, peppermint, and sweet fennel diluted in a carrier oil can provide relief from tummy discomfort.
- Happy mood: A blend of citrus oils like orange, lemon, and grapefruit diluted in a carrier oil can help uplift the mood and promote a positive atmosphere.
- Essential oils for various postpartum needs: Essential oils can assist with various postpartum needs. Some common uses include:
- Afterbirth pains: Essential oils like clary sage and lavender can be used topically to support comfort during afterbirth pains.
- Baby blues: Essential oils such as bergamot and geranium can be diffused or applied topically to uplift the mood and provide emotional support.
- Milk supply: Certain essential oils like fennel or clary sage, when used under the guidance of a lactation consultant, may help support milk supply.
- Perineum spray and healing pads: Lavender, witch hazel, and other soothing oils can be used in DIY perineum sprays or healing pads to promote comfort and healing.
- Energy: Uplifting oils like citrus or peppermint can be used aromatically to provide a natural energy boost for new moms.

ESSENTIAL OILS FOR MOMS OF INFANTS AND TODDLERS

How to Use

Here are some safe and appropriate ways to use essential oils for infants and toddlers:

- Baby massage: Diluted essential oils can be used for gentle massages to promote relaxation and bonding.
- In bath water: Adding a few drops of suitable essential oils to your baby's bathwater can create a soothing and calming experience.
- In a diffuser at bedtime: Diffusing gentle essential oils like lavender or chamomile in your child's bedroom at bedtime can create a peaceful environment and promote better sleep.
- Cold and other viruses: Some essential oils, such as tea tree or eucalyptus, may offer support during times of colds or viral infections. However, it's important to consult with a healthcare professional before using oils for specific conditions and follow their guidance.
- Child navigating strong emotions: Certain essential oils, like citrus oils or lavender, may help soothe and calm an upset or fussy baby. Use them cautiously and observe your baby's response.
- Baby with colic symptoms: Essential oils such as ginger or fennel, when used under the guidance of a healthcare professional, may offer relief for colicky babies.

146 | S. MATHEWS

Remember to always follow proper dilution guidelines and use oils that are safe for babies and children.

Oils to Use

Here are some essential oils that are generally considered safe and suitable for use with babies and children:

- Lavender: It may help promote relaxation and improve sleep quality for both babies and children.
- Chamomile: Known for its gentle and calming effects. It may help soothe irritability, promote relaxation, and support restful sleep.
- Mandarin: It has a sweet and uplifting aroma. It is often used to create a calming and joyful atmosphere, especially during bedtime routines.
- Frankincense: It helps people feel calm and focused. It may help promote a sense of tranquility and emotional balance.
- Tea tree: Known for its antimicrobial properties. It may be used diluted to help address minor skin irritations or as a natural alternative for cleaning purposes.

When using oils on small babies and children, please consult your medical provider for any questions you may have before using essential oils.

Precautions to Take When Massaging a Baby with Essential Oils

If you choose to massage your baby with essential oils, it's important to prioritize their safety and well-being. Here are some precautions to keep in mind:

- Age-appropriate oils: Make use of essential oils that are safe for babies and right for their age. It is generally recommended to use mild and gentle oils such as lavender, chamomile, or mandarin. Avoid using strong or potentially irritating oils on babies.

- Dilution: Essential oils should always be diluted before applying them to your baby's skin. To dilute, use a carrier oil such as sweet almond oil or coconut oil. The recommended dilution ratio for babies is usually one to two droplets of essential oil per ounce of carrier oil.

- Patch test: Do a skin test before you put diluted essential oils on your baby's skin. (Harper, 2016). Apply a small amount of the diluted oil to a small area of their skin, like the inner forearm, and observe for any adverse reactions or sensitivities for at least 24 hours. If any swelling, redness, or irritation occurs, immediately discontinue using it (Harper, 2016).

- Gentle strokes: When massaging your baby, use gentle and light strokes. Avoid applying too much pressure or using vigorous movements.

- Avoid sensitive areas: Be cautious and avoid massaging essential oils on sensitive areas such as the face, genitals, or broken skin. These areas can be more prone to irritation or discomfort.

- Watch for signs of discomfort: Pay attention to your baby's cues and body language during the massage. If they appear uncomfortable, fussy, or show any signs of distress, stop your baby's massage and try again at another time.

- Store oils safely: Safely store essential oils where your children can't reach them to prevent accidental ingestion or spills. It's best to store them in a spot that's not too warm or humid and doesn't get direct sunlight.

Oils to Avoid

When it comes to essential oils for babies and children, some oils have to be avoided due to their potential risks or strong properties. It's important to exercise caution and prioritize the safety of your child. Here are some examples of oils to avoid:

- Peppermint: Peppermint essential oil contains a high concentration of menthol, which can be too intense for babies and young children. It could cause breathing difficulties or skin sensitization.
- Eucalyptus: Eucalyptus essential oil, particularly Eucalyptus globulus, contains a compound called 1,8-cineole, which can potentially harm young children when used in high concentrations or inappropriately. It may cause respiratory distress or irritate the skin. It is advisable to avoid using eucalyptus oil around babies and young children.
- Rosemary: Rosemary essential oil is known for being energizing and contains plenty of camphor. Avoid using rosemary oil on or around infants and young children, as it may cause irritation or overstimulation.
- Wintergreen: Wintergreen essential oil contains high levels of methyl salicylate, which can be toxic if ingested or applied in large amounts. It's important to keep

wintergreen oil out of reach of children and avoid using it on or around them.

- Cinnamon: Cinnamon essential oil is strong and can irritate or make sensitive skin worse, especially in young children.

This is not an exhaustive list; individual sensitivities can vary. Doing thorough research, consulting with a healthcare professional, or seeking advice from a certified aromatherapist before using essential oils with babies or young children is crucial.

THE ADVANTAGES OF USING ESSENTIAL OILS FOR KIDS

Essential oils are extracted from aromatic plants and are entirely natural. Their use for children can offer a range of advantages, including better sleep, decreased anxiety and stress, relief from coughs and colds, and an enhanced immune system. Moreover, particular essential oils possess anti-inflammatory, antibacterial, and antiviral properties that promote overall health and wellness.

Children's essential oils are all-natural products manufactured from fragrant botanicals. They are used all over the world for cleaning, for unwinding, as anti-inflammatories, as stimulants, and even in clinical care.

They have a variety of biological characteristics and are used medicinally, which is why they are growing in popularity. There are several ways that individuals use them nowadays.

Here are some advantages of using essential oils on infants and kids:

Essential oils are one of the best ways to make treatments and creams work more effectively. Let's discuss some advantages of using essential oils for babies and older children.

Helpful Superpowers

During the final stages of recovering from illness, there are some essential oils that can be helpful. Rosehip oil is used most often for these purposes. It can be applied topically to scars daily. Even mothers can get rid of stretch marks by putting rosehip oil on them after their pregnancy. It can even help teenagers keep acne from getting worse (del Carmen Hernandez, 2021).

Keeping Children Calm

When it comes to keeping children calm, one essential oil that can be beneficial is lavender (Lavandula angustifolia). Here are a few suggestions:

- Diffusion: Add a few drops of lavender oil to a diffuser in your child's bedroom or play area to create a peaceful atmosphere.
- Massage: Dilute lavender oil in a carrier oil, such as sweet almond or coconut oil, and gently massage it onto your child's back, chest, or feet. This can help them unwind and relax.
- Bath: Add a few drops of lavender oil to your child's bathwater for a calming and soothing bath experience.

For children under the age of six, it is recommended to use a lower dilution of essential oils (e.g., 0.25%–0.5%) and perform a patch test before use. For specific advice on how to use essential oils with children, always talk to a pediatrician or a trained aromatherapist.

Don't forget that every child is different, and their reactions to essential oils may be different too. It's important to observe your child's reactions and discontinue use if any signs of irritation or discomfort occur.

Antibacterial Properties

Coconut oil is preferable due to its antibacterial properties, while tea tree oil is also beneficial as it has antibacterial, antimicrobial, and anti-inflammatory properties (del Carmen Hernandez, 2021). These oils help treat cuts, scratches, burns, and insect bites and can also be used as an insect repellent. Additionally, basil and citronella oils are also effective in keeping bugs away. However, it is important to note that these oils should not be applied to babies under six months old.

Treating Headaches and Insomnia

There are a number of essential oils that can possibly reduce migraines. According to studies conducted by European Neurology, using lavender essential oil by inhaling it can be a dependable and safe method to alleviate migraines (del Carmen Hernandez, 2021). According to Blair (2020), using peppermint essential oil can reduce headaches in children over the age of two and a half. There are several types of oils that can be used to assist children in falling asleep. If you have trouble sleeping,

152 | S. MATHEWS

lavender may be able to help. The calming properties of lavender make it an effective treatment for insomnia. Simply adding two or three drops of lavender essential oil to a vapor diffuser can have a powerfully relaxing effect.

If your child struggles with nighttime terrors, you can try diffusing Roman chamomile to calm them. Marjoram has anxiety-reducing, hyperactivity-reducing, and stress-reducing properties and a pleasant scent (del Carmen Hernandez, 2021).

Treatment for Panic and Anxiety

If you want to help children feel better and less anxious, you can use sweet orange oil, basil, lavender, frankincense, and chamomile. These oils have a calming effect on their nerves. To make them feel refreshed and relaxed, you can also use peppermint oil.

Nausea and Tiredness

When it comes to addressing feelings of nausea and combating tiredness, essential oils can provide natural and soothing support. Blair (2020) suggests ginger, peppermint, and mandarin oil as options for reducing nausea in children over two and a half years old.

The Moisturizing Effect of Essential Oils

Did you know that avocado essential oil is one of the most hydrating oils and a popular choice for treating dry skin? It's packed with vitamin A, vitamin E, and healthy fatty acids that are great for your skin. Another moisturizing oil is lavender oil, which can also aid in the healthy regeneration of damaged skin (del Carmen Hernandez, 2021).

Cradle Cap Treatment

If you are experiencing skin conditions marked by desquamation, such as cradle cap, scalp psoriasis, or seborrheic dermatitis, it is recommended to use almond oil to eliminate the scales.

Flu or Cold Treatment

If your child has a cold and has trouble sleeping at night, using fragrant essential oils such as lavender might help relieve their symptoms and give them a calm night of sleep. Oils like menthol, camphor, and eucalyptus work well. Chamomile oil and melaleuca oil have antiviral properties that may be beneficial.

Gas or Stomach Cramps

So many essential oils have antispasmodic results. To put it simply, they alleviate the pain that results from stomach contractions. There are several essential oils that can be helpful, including ginger, chamomile, and lavender. Peppermint essential oil is particularly effective in supporting healthy digestion by promoting proper stomach and intestinal function.

Always consult a medical provider to seek advice or consultation before using essential oils on any of the above physical symptoms.

IMPORTANT SAFETY TIPS FOR USING ESSENTIAL OILS WITH CHILDREN

When it comes to using essential oils safely, there are a few options to consider. You can apply them topically to your children's skin or use an aroma stick, which acts like an inhaler. However, be cautious not to overuse the diffuser and avoid using it in crowded areas to prevent overwhelming others. If you prefer a more personal experience, an aroma stick is a great option for inhaling the scent.

To avoid skin irritation in your child, it is best to dilute oils with a carrier oil before applying. It is important to keep in mind the appropriate dosage for each age range to ensure safety. You can follow the guidelines provided by Blair (2020) to keep your kids feeling fresh and comfortable:

- 3–24 months: 0.25%–0.5%
- Two to six years: up to 2%
- Six to fifteen years: 1.5%–3%
- Older than 15 years: 2.5%–5%

If your child experiences any negative symptoms, such as a skin rash, headaches, or difficulty breathing, it is important to contact your doctor immediately. While essential oils may be enjoyable, they are not a replacement for expert medical attention.

AROMATHERAPY FOR TEENS AND MOMS

Using aromatherapy is a natural and helpful way for mothers with teenage children to improve their well-being. Aromatherapy can be helpful for moms of teens by using essential oils to address specific concerns and promote relaxation. Let's look more closely at the different ways it can be used:

- Skin troubles: Essential oils like tea tree, lavender, and frankincense can help address common skin issues that teenagers may face, such as acne or blemishes. These oils possess antibacterial and soothing properties that can support skin health.
- Homework, study, and focus: Rosemary, peppermint, and lemon essential oils are recognized for boosting concentration, mental clarity, and focus. Diffusing these oils or using them in a personal inhaler while studying or doing homework can create a conducive environment for better focus and productivity.
- Period pain and PMS: Essential oils like clary sage and lavender can help ease menstrual discomfort and alleviate symptoms associated with premenstrual syndrome (PMS). You can apply these oils to your skin, mix them with a carrier oil, or put them in a warm bath to help you relax and feel better.
- Getting up in the morning: Orange, grapefruit, and lemon oils are known for their uplifting and energizing qualities. Inhaling these oils or using them in a morning shower gel or lotion can help moms and teens feel refreshed and energized to start the day.

156 | S. MATHEWS

- Sleep and relaxation: Essential oils such as lavender, chamomile, and ylang-ylang have calming and soothing effects that can promote better sleep and relaxation. Diffusing these oils in the bedroom or using them in a bedtime routine can create a serene atmosphere and support a restful night's sleep.
- Stress and mild anxiety: Essential oils like bergamot, clary sage, and frankincense have been known to help reduce stress and mild anxiety. These oils can be used in diffusers, inhalers, or diluted in carrier oils for topical application to provide a sense of calm and relaxation.
- Sports and exercise: Essential oils such as peppermint and eucalyptus have invigorating and cooling properties that can be beneficial for sports and exercise. These oils can be added to a post-workout massage oil or used in a refreshing spray to provide a cooling sensation and support muscle recovery.
- Confidence and courage: Essential oils like jasmine, rosemary, and cedarwood are known for their uplifting and confidence-boosting properties. These oils can be used in personal aromatherapy inhalers or diluted in carrier oils for topical application to enhance self-assurance and courage.

AROMATHERAPY FOR OLDER MOTHERS, GRANDMOTHERS, AND WOMEN

Aromatherapy can be a valuable tool for grandmothers to manage various physical and emotional concerns. This approach promotes relaxation, relieves pain, and improves overall well-being using natural and holistic methods. Let's explore how aromatherapy can benefit older mothers, grandmothers and women by addressing their specific needs.

Uses

- Anxiety and depression: Lavender, bergamot, and chamomile are all essential oils that can help calm and balance your mood. These oils may help calm people down and make them feel better emotionally if they are anxious or depressed.
- Dementia or Alzheimer's disease: Aromatherapy may be beneficial in supporting individuals with dementia or Alzheimer's disease. Some essential oils, including lemon, rosemary, and peppermint, can enhance cognitive function, improve memory, and increase alertness.
- Fighting infections: Some essential oils possess antibacterial and antiviral properties, making them useful in fighting common infections like colds, coughs, flu, and blocked sinuses. Eucalyptus, tea tree, and lemon oils can be beneficial for supporting the respiratory system and boosting immunity.
- Boosting memory: Essential oils like rosemary and peppermint have been associated with improved memory and concentration. Diffusing these oils or using them in a personal inhaler during cognitive tasks or studying may enhance focus and recall.

- Improving overall mood: Did you know that aromatherapy is an effective way to improve your mood and create a positive atmosphere? Citrus oils like orange, lemon, and grapefruit, as well as floral oils such as ylang-ylang and geranium, are particularly effective at enhancing your mood. Give them a try!

Massage Blends for Pain Relief

- For arthritis: Essential oils like ginger, frankincense, and lavender can be used in massage blends to help alleviate pain and stiffness associated with arthritis because of their pain-relieving and anti-inflammatory benefits.
- Dry and cracked skin: Certain essential oils like lavender, geranium, and chamomile have hydrating and soothing properties that can help nourish dry and cracked skin. Incorporating them into massage blends or skincare products can provide relief and promote healthier skin.
- General stiffness and sore areas: Aromatherapy massage blends containing oils like marjoram, peppermint, and eucalyptus can help relieve general stiffness and target specific sore areas because of their pain-relieving and anti-inflammatory benefits.

Sleep Problems

Essential oils such as lavender, chamomile, and sandalwood are renowned for their calming and sedative effects. Diffusing these oils in the bedroom or using them in a bedtime routine can promote relaxation and improve sleep quality. If you like to wind down before bedtime. use a carrier oil and combine it with vetiver oil. The deep and earthy scent helps relax and ensures a restful night's sleep.

Precautions for Grandmothers

By incorporating aromatherapy into their daily routines, grandmothers can experience the potential benefits of improved well-being, reduced pain, enhanced relaxation, and a greater sense of calm and joy in their lives. It's essential for grandmothers to take certain precautions when using aromatherapy. Diluting essential oils properly, using appropriate concentrations, and considering any existing health conditions or medications are crucial aspects to ensuring safe usage. If you have specific health concerns or allergies, it is best to talk to a healthcare professional or a qualified aromatherapist.

In this chapter, we discussed how essential oils can be beneficial for pregnant mothers, offering insights into their safe usage during pregnancy and addressing specific concerns such as morning sickness, postpartum recovery, and relaxation. We then moved on to exploring the use of essential oils for new moms, focusing on skincare, postpartum recovery, and promoting a soothing environment for both the mother and the newborn. We provided information on how to safely use essential oils for infants and toddlers, including tips on precautions, appropriate oils, and different ways to apply them. In addition, we talked about how aromatherapy can help mothers and teenagers with skincare problems, improve concentration, improve emotional health, and address sports-related issues.

In the next chapter, we will explore the concept of chemical-free living by integrating essential oils into our cleaning and home care practices. We will explore how these natural and versatile oils can replace harmful chemicals and provide effective solutions for cleaning, disinfecting, and creating a healthier environment for ourselves and our families. Get ready to discover how the power of essential oils can transform your home into a safe and chemical-free haven.

7

TOXIC TO TRANQUIL—
TRANSFORM YOUR HOME WITH
ESSENTIAL OILS

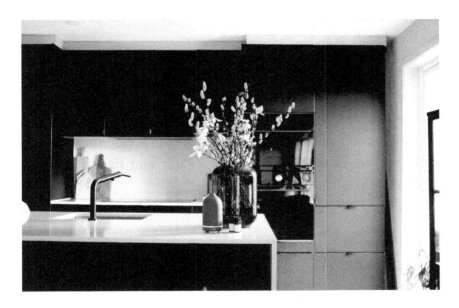

Our homes ought to be a place of refuge where we feel secure and shielded. However, our homes are filled with a wide range of everyday products that contain harmful chemicals. Cleaning supplies, air fresheners, personal care products, and carpeting can release toxic substances into the air we breathe. These chemicals can contribute to indoor air pollution and have been linked to various health issues such as respiratory problems, allergies, skin irritations, hormonal disruptions, and other serious health conditions.

Essential oils provide a safe and efficient method for cleaning and maintaining our living spaces, eliminating the necessity for detrimental substances. These oils are derived from plants and possess powerful properties that can disinfect, deodorize, and provide various therapeutic benefits. By harnessing the aromatic and antimicrobial properties of essential oils, we can create a chemical-free environment that promotes both cleanliness and well-being.

Let's discuss practical tips and recipes for incorporating essential oils into our cleaning and home care routines. From all-purpose cleaners and air fresheners to laundry detergents and personal care products, we will explore how essential oils can replace toxic chemicals, ensuring a safer and healthier living space for ourselves and our loved ones.

HOW TO USE ESSENTIAL OILS FOR A CHEMICAL-FREE HOME

Get ready to transform your home into a haven of wellness and sustainability by embracing the power of essential oils. Transitioning to a chemical-free home is an important step towards safeguarding our health and well-being and caring for our environment. Here are some steps and tips to help you create a chemical-free home:

- Educate yourself: Start by educating yourself about the harmful effects of chemicals generally found in household products. Understand the potential risks associated with these chemicals and their impact on your health and the environment.
- Clean out toxic products: Begin by decluttering your home and getting rid of products that contain toxic chemicals. This includes cleaning supplies, air fresheners, personal care products, and pesticides. Make sure you follow the required regulations when disposing of these products.
- Opt for natural cleaning solutions: Embrace natural alternatives for cleaning your home. Essential oils such as lemon, tea tree, and lavender have powerful cleaning properties and can be used to make homemade cleaners. If you want to clean with natural products, baking soda, vinegar, and hydrogen peroxide have all been shown to work well.
- Choose non-toxic personal care products: Check the labels of personal care products, including soaps, shampoos, lotions, and cosmetics. Look for products that are free from parabens, phthalates, sulfates, and artificial fragrances. Consider making your own natural skincare and beauty products using essential oils and simple ingredients.
- Purify your indoor air: Improve the air quality in your home by using natural air purifiers such as houseplants,

salt lamps, and air-purifying essential oils like eucalyptus and peppermint. It's an excellent idea to open your windows often to let fresh air flow through your home.

- Create a chemical-free nursery: If you have a baby or young children, create a chemical-free environment in their nursery. Use organic bedding, non-toxic toys, and natural cleaning products to reduce their exposure to harmful chemicals.
- Natural pest control measures: Instead of using chemicals to get rid of pests inside and outside your home, it's better to use natural methods. Essential oils like peppermint, citronella, and neem oil can be effective in repelling insects.

By following these steps and embracing a chemical-free lifestyle, you can create a healthier and more sustainable home environment for yourself and future generations.

ESSENTIAL OILS FOR HOUSEHOLD CLEANING PURPOSES

Essential oils can be used to clean because they are good at killing bacteria, viruses, and fungi. They can help kill germs, remove stains, and freshen the air without the use of harsh chemicals. Here are a few ideas for how you can use essential oils to clean. Essential oils can be used to create homemade cleaning solutions that are effective and safe. They can be used in various cleaning applications, such as floor cleaning, kitchen sink scrubbing, all-purpose cleaning, and air cleaning. Essential oils mixed with other natural ingredients like vinegar, baking soda, or castile soap can be used to make cleaning products that work well.

There are several essential oils that are particularly beneficial for cleaning. Lemon, lavender, tea tree, eucalyptus, peppermint, and orange are some popular choices. These oils have strong cleaning properties and add a pleasant fragrance to your cleaning products.

- Vacuum cleaning: Drip some essential oil into your vacuum machine to make your carpets smell fresh again.
- Kitchen sink scrub: Make a paste of liquid castile soap, baking soda, and a few drops of essential oil to use as a kitchen sink scrub.
- All-purpose cleaning solutions: Combine essential oils with vinegar or water in a spray bottle.
- Air fresheners: Essential oils can also be diffused or added to homemade air fresheners to clean and purify the air in your home.
- Pest repellent: Rosemary oil is not only antimicrobial but also an effective insect repellent. Properly dilute it with water in a spray container.
- You can use it in areas where bugs gather, such as kitchens for ants or porches and garages for wasps.
- DIY hacks: In addition to cleaning, essential oils have many other household uses. They can be used to freshen laundry, eliminate odors, remove sticky residues, and more. With a little creativity, you can find

numerous DIY hacks that incorporate essential oils into your daily household tasks.

Kitchen Cleaning Recipes

When you use essential oils to clean your kitchen, you can avoid using chemicals and enjoy the aroma too. Here are various ways you can use essential oils for kitchen cleaning:

- Kitchen diffuser blends: You can create your own kitchen diffuser blends by combining essential oils like lemon, orange, or peppermint. Just pour a few droplets of your favorite essential oil into a diffuser and let the smell fill your kitchen.
- Cleaning counters: Create a homemade countertop cleaner by mixing water, white vinegar, and a few drops of essential oils such as lemon, tea tree, or lavender. Combine everything into a spray bottle and use it to clean the kitchen counters.
- Fridge deodorizer: To naturally deodorize your fridge, place a few drops of essential oils like lemon, eucalyptus, or mint on a cotton ball and put it in a small dish. Keep the dish inside the fridge to freshen the air.
- Air freshener: Make your own air freshener spray by combining distilled water and a few drops of essential oils such as lemon, lavender, or citrus blends. Combine the ingredients in a spray bottle and use it to freshen the air in your kitchen.
- Floor cleaner: Add a few drops of essential oils like lemon, tea tree, or pine to a bucket of warm water,

along with your preferred natural floor cleaner. Use this solution to mop your kitchen floors, leaving behind a pleasant scent.

- Washing dishes: Add a few drops of essential oils like lemon, lavender, or citrus blends to your dish soap or dishwasher for a pleasant fragrance and potential antibacterial benefits.
- Refresh the drawers: Place cotton balls infused with essential oils such as lavender, cedarwood, or citrus blends in kitchen drawers to keep them smelling fresh.
- Garbage deodorizer: Add a few drops of essential oils like lemon, tea tree, or eucalyptus to a cotton ball and place it at the bottom of the garbage bin to help neutralize odors.
- Steam clean the microwave: Add a few drops of lemon or citrus essential oil to a microwave-safe bowl filled with water. Heat the bowl in the microwave for a few minutes to create steam that will help loosen food splatters and freshen the microwave.

By incorporating these practical tips, you can effectively use essential oils in your kitchen cleaning routine to create a chemical-free and pleasantly scented environment.

Bathroom Cleaning Tips

Here is some practical information regarding the use of essential oils in bathroom cleaning:

- Refresh your bathrooms with essential oils: Add a few drops of your favorite essential oils, such as lavender, eucalyptus, or citrus blends, to a diffuser in your bathroom to create a fresh and inviting atmosphere.

- Bathroom diffuser blends: Make a scrub for the kitchen sink by mixing liquid castile soap, baking soda, and some essential oil of your choice into a paste.
- Prevent bad odors: Use essential oils with natural deodorizing properties, such as lemon, tea tree, or lavender, to help eliminate unpleasant odors in the bathroom. Simply add a few drops to a cotton ball and place it in the bathroom to freshen the air.
- Best essential oils for bathroom: Essential oils like eucalyptus, tea tree, peppermint, and lavender are generally recommended for their cleansing and deodorizing properties in the bathroom.
- Toilet cleaner: Make a homemade toilet cleaner by combining baking soda, white vinegar, and a few drops of essential oils like tea tree or lemon. Apply the mixture to the toilet bowl, scrub, and then flush for a fresh and clean result.
- No-scrub toilet bowl cleaner: Create a no-scrub toilet bowl cleaner by adding a few drops of essential oils like tea tree, lemon, or eucalyptus to the inside of the toilet tank. The essential oils will mix with the water and help keep the bowl clean with each flush.
- Bathroom sink, grout, and tub cleaner: Mix baking soda, water, and a few drops of essential oils like tea tree or lemon to form a paste. Use the paste to scrub sinks, grout lines, and tub surfaces, then rinse with water for a sparkling clean result.

- Bathroom spray: Make your own natural bathroom spray by combining water, witch hazel, and a few drops of essential oils like lavender, eucalyptus, or citrus blends. Use this spray to freshen the air and surfaces in your bathroom.
- Anti-fungal spray: To combat mold and mildew in the bathroom, create an anti-fungal spray by mixing water, white vinegar, and a few drops of essential oils like scotch pine, spearmint, tea tree oil, or grapefruit seed extract. Spray it on the affected areas and let it sit for a while before wiping clean.
- Shower cleaner: Mix water, white vinegar, and a few drops of essential oils like tea tree or eucalyptus in a spray bottle. You can use this solution to clean and disinfect your shower, including the tiles and glass. You can also mix 30 droplets of bitter orange essential oil, a quarter cup of lemon juice, and a quarter cup of baking soda in a container. Mix well. Apply the mixture to the shower or tub and let it sit for about 15 minutes. Scrub with a scouring pad to remove dirt and stains. Rinse thoroughly with water.

By utilizing these practical tips, you can effectively incorporate essential oils into your bathroom cleaning routine, promoting a clean, fresh, and chemical-free environment.

ESSENTIAL OILS AND YOUR LAUNDRY

Will Adding Essential Oils to Your Laundry Work?

Yes, you could really add essential oils to your laundry to give your garments a nice smell and maybe get some of their aromatherapy benefits. Essential oils can give your laundry a natural scent without having to use the chemicals that are in most detergents and fabric softeners.

Which Oils Should You Use?

There are many different essential oils you can use in your laundry, depending on your personal preferences. Popular choices include lavender, lemon, eucalyptus, tea tree, and peppermint. Lavender offers a calming scent; lemon provides a fresh and citrusy aroma; eucalyptus has a refreshing and invigorating fragrance; tea tree offers natural disinfecting properties; and peppermint gives off a cooling and energizing scent.

Oils for Disinfecting Laundry

If you want to add disinfecting properties to your laundry, consider using essential oils such as tea tree, eucalyptus, or lavender. The antimicrobial properties possessed by these oils can assist in eradicating bacteria and fungi.

Do Essential Oils Ruin Clothes?

When used properly, essential oils should not ruin clothes. However, it's important to dilute the essential oils before adding them to your laundry to prevent any potential staining or damage. Be cautious with dark-colored or delicate fabrics, and always do a patch test on a small, inconspicuous area before using essential oils on your clothes.

How to Use Essential Oils in Your Laundry

Several methods exist for integrating essential oils into your laundry routine:

- In your washer: Add a few droplets of essential oil to the detergent compartment or directly into the drum before starting the wash cycle. This allows the oils to infuse with the water and distribute evenly among the clothes. Lavender, grapefruit, rosemary, cedarwood, and lemon oil are all great options.
- Wool dryer balls: Add a few droplets of essential oil to your wool dryer balls. It can help decrease static and soften your fabrics during the drying process. The essential oils will release their aroma as the balls tumble with the clothes. Personally, I like using lemongrass oil, but you may also want to consider trying lemon, peppermint, or lavender oils.

Essential Oils Laundry Blends

- Blending a laundry detergent: You'll need two cups of soap flakes or grated soap bars, half a cup of baking soda, a full cup of washing soda, and a teaspoon of your favorite essential oil or essential oil combination (20 Best Homemade Laundry Detergent, 2023). Chemical-free fabric softener: Commercial fabric softeners often contain synthetic chemicals that can be harsh on the skin and the environment. However, you can create a chemical-free alternative using ingredients like vinegar and essential oils. Simply mix equal parts of water and white vinegar, then add a few drops of your preferred essential oil. Lavender, chamomile, or citrus scents work well for fabric softening. Store this mixture in a spray bottle and lightly spritz it onto your clothes before transferring them to the dryer. The vinegar helps to soften the fabric, while the essential oils provide a delightful fragrance.

- Homemade linen spray: A homemade linen spray is an excellent way to freshen up your linens, curtains, or upholstery or for air freshening. To make your own linen spray, combine water and a few droplets of essential oil in a spray bottle. Lavender, rose, or chamomile essential oils are popular choices for creating a relaxing and soothing ambiance. Spritz the mixture onto your fabrics or into the air to enjoy the refreshing scent.

- Pre-wash stain remover: Dealing with tough stains on your clothes before washing them can be a challenge. Fortunately, you can create a pre-wash stain remover using simple ingredients found in your kitchen pantry. One effective option is to mix equal parts of liquid dish soap and hydrogen peroxide. Apply this mixture directly to the stain and gently rub it in. Let it sit for a few minutes before laundering the garment as usual. This homemade stain remover helps to break down and lift stubborn stains, preparing your clothes for a thorough clean.

Our sense of smell has a significant impact on our well-being, affecting our mood, mindset, and environment. By adding the right fragrances to our living spaces, we can create a comfortable and inviting atmosphere that suits our personal choices and enhances our daily lives.

In the next chapter, we will explore a variety of fragrances and how they can be used throughout the home. From revitalizing scents to calming aromas, we will discover how fragrances can transform our homes into tranquil havens. First, we will delve into essential oils and their unique properties. We will learn about the most popular oils, their therapeutic benefits, and how to incorporate them into our daily lives. Whether you prefer the uplifting scent of citrus, the serene aroma of lavender, or the grounding fragrance of sandalwood, we will explore the versatility of these oils and their transformative effects on our living spaces.

8

YOUR FRAGRANCE SWATCHES

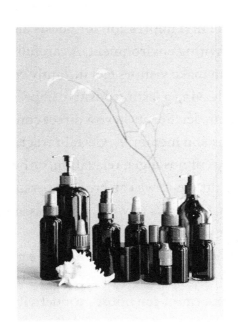

S electing the appropriate fragrance for your home is crucial to establishing a pleasant and peaceful environment. Home scents are more than just a cover-up for bad smells. They can evoke emotions, create an atmosphere, and improve our well-being. Let's explore the importance of scents in our households:

- Creating an inviting ambiance: The scent of our home sets the first impression for guests and creates a warm and inviting environment. A carefully chosen fragrance can make visitors feel instantly comfortable and at ease, leaving a lasting positive impression. The scent of our home sets the first impression for guests and creates a warm and inviting environment. A carefully chosen fragrance can make visitors feel instantly comfortable and at ease, leaving a lasting positive impression.
- Emotional impact: Scents have a direct connection to our emotions and memories. Certain fragrances can evoke feelings of nostalgia, relaxation, or happiness. Using the right scent, we can create a personal sanctuary that helps us unwind, de-stress, and find solace in our homes.
- Mood enhancement: Fragrances have the power to influence our mood and mindset. Energizing scents like citrus or peppermint can boost productivity and focus. At the same time, soothing aromas like lavender or chamomile can promote relaxation and better sleep. By selecting scents that align with our desired mood, we

can transform our living spaces into supportive environments for our daily activities.

- Personal expression: The scents we choose for our homes reflect our preferences and can be an extension of our identity. Whether it's a crisp, clean scent for a minimalist aesthetic or a warm, cozy fragrance for a rustic atmosphere, home scents allow us to showcase our style and create an environment that resonates with us.

- Well-being and stress relief: Certain scents, such as lavender or eucalyptus, have been known for their therapeutic properties. They can help reduce stress and anxiety, promote relaxation, and create a calming environment. It can help us relax and de-stress from our daily routine.

- Association with cleanliness: Pleasant scents are often associated with cleanliness and freshness. Using fragrances in cleaning products or air fresheners can create the impression of a clean and well-maintained home, even if that may not always be the case. This association can contribute to a positive overall perception of the space.

21 ESSENTIAL OILS YOU NEED IN YOUR CUPBOARD

These essential oils can be used for various purposes, including promoting relaxation, reducing stress and anxiety, improving sleep, supporting healthy respiratory function, soothing sore muscles, and promoting overall well-being. Each oil has its unique properties and benefits, allowing you to create a personalized aromatic experience in your home.

Explore this list of 21 essential oils to enhance your home environment:

- Bergamot
- Cedarwood
- Clary sage
- Eucalyptus
- Frankincense
- Geranium
- Ginger
- Jasmine
- Lavender
- Lemon
- Marjoram
- Neroli
- Patchouli
- Peppermint
- Roman chamomile
- Rose
- Sandalwood
- Tea tree
- Vetiver
- Ylang-ylang

Scan the QR code at the end of this book to get your free copy of the Essential 21 Oils Guide.

Five DIY Essential Oil Recipes

Soothing Muscle Rub

The soothing muscle tub is specifically designed to target those areas that need extra care and attention. Whether it's your shoulders, back, legs, or any other area of discomfort, massage a small amount of the rub onto the affected muscles and let the soothing blend work its magic.

Ingredients

- Two tablespoons of coconut oil (carrier)
- Five droplets (drops) of eucalyptus oil
- Five droplets of lavender oil
- Five droplets of peppermint oil

Directions

To get started, warm up the coconut oil using either a microwave or double boiler until it becomes liquid. After that, let it cool for a short while before mixing in the essential oils. Stir well, and pour the mixture into a small container. Apply the rub to sore muscles and joints for a soothing effect.

Cooling After-Sun Gel

Experience instant relief and nourishment for your sun-kissed skin with the cooling after-sun gel. Formulated with soothing aloe vera and cooling cucumber extract, this refreshing gel will soothe and hydrate your skin after a day in the sun, leaving you feeling rejuvenated and ready for more summer adventures.

Ingredients

- A quarter cup (4 tablespoons) of aloe vera gel (carrier)
- One tablespoon (180 droplets) of jojoba oil
- Five droplets of peppermint oil
- Five droplets of lavender oil

Directions

In a tiny bowl, combine the aloe vera gel and jojoba oil. Add your essential oils and blend them well. Transfer the mixture to an airtight jar or bottle. Apply the gel to sun-exposed skin for a cooling and soothing effect.

Refreshing Citrus Body Scrub

Indulge in the invigorating experience of our refreshing citrus body scrub. Packed with zesty citrus essential oils and natural exfoliants, this revitalizing scrub will gently buff away dead skin cells, leaving your skin feeling refreshed, smooth, and glowing with a burst of citrus-infused energy.

Ingredients

- One cup (or 16 tablespoons) of granulated sugar
- A quarter cup (4 tablespoons) of coconut oil
- Ten droplets of orange oil
- Five droplets of lemon oil
- Five droplets of grapefruit oil

- Five droplets of lemon oil

Directions

Blend the sugar and coconut oil. Add the essential oils and stir thoroughly. Transfer the mixture to a jar with a tight lid. Apply your body scrub while in the shower by gently massaging it onto damp skin in circular movements. Rinse off for refreshed and smooth skin.

Revitalizing Peppermint Foot Soak

Treat your tired feet to a luxurious and rejuvenating experience with our revitalizing peppermint foot soak recipe. Infused with the refreshing aroma of peppermint essential oil, this soothing foot soak will help relieve fatigue, soften rough skin, and leave your feet feeling cool, revitalized, and ready to take on the world.

Ingredients

- One cup (or 16 tablespoons) of Epsom salt
- A quarter cup (4 tablespoons) of baking soda
- Ten droplets of peppermint essential oil
- One tablespoon of carrier oil (such as almond oil or coconut oil)
- Optional: fresh or alternatively dried peppermint leaves (for added fragrance)

Directions

Mix the Epsom salt and baking soda together in a bowl, ensuring that they are thoroughly combined. Add the almond or coconut carrier oil and the peppermint oil and carrier to the dry mixture. Mix well until the oils are evenly distributed. If desired, crush a few dried peppermint leaves or add fresh mint leaves to the mixture for an extra burst of fragrance. Store the foot soak mixture in a container with a tight-fitting lid. To use, fill a basin or tub with warm water and add 1/4 to 1/2 cup of the foot soak mixture. Stir the water to dissolve the mixture and create a refreshing foot-soak solution. Soak your feet in the mixture for 15–20 minutes, allowing the peppermint and Epsom salt to relax and revitalize your tired feet. Once you are done soaking your feet, wash them with warm water and gently dry them by patting them with a towel. Follow up with a moisturizer or foot cream for added hydration and softness.

Energizing Citrus Room Spray

This energizing citrus room spray is a great way to add a zesty and rejuvenating aroma to your home or office. It's perfect for creating a vibrant and energizing environment.

Ingredients

- Half a cup (8 tablespoons) of distilled water
- Two tablespoons of vodka or rubbing alcohol (which acts as a preservative)
- 15 droplets of sweet orange essential oil
- Ten droplets of lemon oil
- Five droplets of grapefruit oil

Directions

In a small spray bottle, combine the distilled water and vodka or rubbing alcohol. Essential oils like sweet orange, lemon, and grapefruit should be added now. Put a tight lid on the spray container and give it a good shake to mix the contents.

YOUR FRAGRANCE GUIDE FOR SCENTS IN THE HOME

Elevate your living space with your own fragrance guide for captivating scents in the home. Diffusers, room sprays, and incense are popular options for adding fragrance to your home. Diffusers, both reed and essential oil, offer flameless options with different methods of dispersing scent. For a quick and efficient way to mask unwanted smells, room sprays and gel beads are great choices. They can provide a pleasant aroma in no time.

Creating a pleasant and inviting ambiance in your home goes beyond just visual aesthetics. Choosing the right fragrances can elevate the atmosphere and evoke different moods in each room. Here's a fragrance guide to help you determine which scents to use where in your home:

- Living room: In most homes, the living room is where the majority of people gather. Choose scents that are warm and inviting, like vanilla, cinnamon, or amber, to create a nice and cozy space. These fragrances can help promote relaxation and a sense of warmth, making them ideal for entertaining guests or unwinding after a long day.

- Bedroom: For a good night's sleep, it's important to make the bedroom a calm and relaxing place. Choose fragrances like lavender, chamomile, or jasmine, known for their relaxing properties. These scents can help reduce stress and anxiety, setting the stage for a peaceful night's sleep.
- Kitchen: The kitchen is often filled with various aromas from cooking and food preparation. To combat any lingering odors and keep the space smelling fresh, go for citrus-based scents like lemon or orange. These fragrances are invigorating and can help create a clean and uplifting atmosphere.
- Bathroom: For the bathroom, a clean and refreshing scent is desirable. Look for crisp and light fragrances such as eucalyptus, mint, or sea breeze. These scents can provide a sense of freshness and cleanliness, transforming your bathroom into a spa-like oasis.
- Home office: In a home office, it's essential to foster focus and concentration. Opt for energizing scents like rosemary, peppermint, or citrus blends. These fragrances can help stimulate the mind and enhance productivity, making them perfect for a workspace.
- Entryway: The entryway sets the first impression for your home. Choose welcoming scents like fresh linen, green tea, or a subtle floral bouquet. These fragrances create an inviting atmosphere and greet guests with a pleasant aroma as they walk inside.

Experiment with different scents and adjust according to your taste and the overall mood you wish to create in each room. It's also important to avoid overpowering fragrances and maintain a subtle balance to ensure a pleasant experience for everyone in your home.

YOUR QUICK REFERENCE ESSENTIAL OILS DICTIONARY

- Bergamot: A citrus essential oil known for its uplifting and mood-enhancing properties and for relieving skin irritations. It is often used in aromatherapy to help people feel less anxious and calm down.
- Cedarwood: A woody and earthy essential oil with a warm and comforting aroma. It is generally used for its calming properties, promoting relaxation, and supporting a healthy respiratory system.
- Chamomile: It calms, soothes, and helps you sleep.
- Clary sage: Oil extracted from the clary sage plant, used for its calming and balancing properties in aromatherapy. Stress, menstruation pain, and lack of sleep can all benefit from its use.
- Eucalyptus: This oil is known for having a scent that is both refreshing and energizing. It is often used for respiratory support, soothing sore muscles, and promoting a clear mind.
- Frankincense: An essential oil with the fragrance and consistency of resinous wood. It is often used for its

grounding and centering properties, as well as for skincare and meditation practices.

- Geranium: An aromatic flower oil that is both pleasant and uplifting to the senses. It is often used to balance emotions, support healthy skin, and repel insects.
- Ginger: A spicy and warming essential oil with a distinctively pungent aroma. It is known for its digestive properties, soothing muscle discomfort, and promoting healthy circulation.
- Grapefruit: A citrus essential oil with a tangy and uplifting aroma. It is generally used to boost mood, support digestion, and enhance skin health.
- Jasmine: An essential oil distilled from the jasmine plant's blooms. It smells deliciously exotic and is packed with power. It has a sweet, exotic aroma and is highly prized for its aphrodisiac qualities and ability to uplift the mood.
- Lavender: It is calming and soothing and promotes relaxation.
- Lemon: It is uplifting and purifying and enhances mood.
- Lemongrass: A fresh and citrusy essential oil known for its energizing and revitalizing properties. It is often used to relieve muscle tension, repel insects, and promote a sense of balance.
- Marjoram: An herbaceous essential oil with a warm and spicy fragrance. It is valued for its calming effects, promoting restful sleep, and soothing tired muscles.
- Myrrh: An earthy and resinous essential oil with a warm and comforting scent. It is highly valued for its

grounding and spiritual properties, as well as its ability to support skin health.

- Neroli: The blooms of the bitter orange tree are used to produce a flowery essential oil. It has a sweet and delicate scent and is often used for its calming, uplifting, and skin-nourishing properties.
- Patchouli: An essential oil with a musky, earthy aroma that evokes thoughts of hippie culture. It is known for its grounding and balancing properties, as well as its skin-regenerating effects.
- Peppermint: A cooling and refreshing essential oil with a minty aroma. It is widely recognized for its invigorating and digestive benefits, as well as its ability to promote focus and clarity.
- Rose: A luxurious floral essential oil with a romantic and exquisite scent. It is highly prized for its skin-rejuvenating properties, emotional balancing effects, and promotion of feelings of love and well-being.
- Rosemary: An essential oil distilled from aromatic herbs; has a warm, woodsy aroma. It is generally used to stimulate the mind by improving memory and concentration, supporting respiratory health, and promoting a healthy scalp and hair growth.
- Sandalwood: A woody essential oil with a warm, exotic scent. It is commonly used in spiritual and meditative practices because of its relaxing and centering properties.
- Tea tree: A powerful essential oil with antimicrobial properties. It is generally used for its purifying and

188 | S. MATHEWS

cleansing effects, particularly in skincare and hair care products.

- Vetiver: A deep, earthy essential oil derived from the roots of the vetiver grass. Because of its calming and focusing effects, it is frequently employed in religious and meditation rituals.
- Ylang-ylang: A floral essential oil with a rich and exotic fragrance. It is highly sought-after for its calming effects, mood-boosting qualities, and sensual enhancement.

I WOULD LOVE TO HEAR FROM YOU!

Your feedback and support have played an instrumental role in extending the reach of my book, "Aromatherapy for Self Care," to a diverse audience of women, mothers, grandmothers, and beyond.

I would be deeply appreciative if you could spare a moment to share your insights and impressions about my book.

I invite you to kindly consider leaving a review on Amazon once it becomes available. Thank you wholeheartedly for your unwavering support, which continues to inspire and drive my passion for aromatherapy and self-care.

Scan the QR code below

CONCLUSION

Thank you for reading *Aromatherapy for Self-Care*. Writing this book has been an inspiration for my personal healing journey. I hope this book has provided helpful insights about aromatherapy and inspired you to incorporate essential oils into your routine for better health and wellness.

In this book, we have delved into the many advantages of essential oils and how they can be used for self-care. Essential oils can help with relaxation, stress relief, physical well-being, and creating a calming atmosphere at home. They are effective tools for taking care of oneself.

Always remember that taking care of yourself and prioritizing your health are important. You can achieve this by using essential oils in your daily life. This proactive step will not only benefit you but also your loved ones.

As you continue your journey, always prioritize safety by choosing high-quality essential oils and seeking guidance from qualified professionals when needed. Explore various blends and applications to find what resonates best with you.

I sincerely wish you the best on your aromatherapy journey. May you find joy, balance, and rejuvenation as you explore the world of essential oils. Your self-care journey is personal and transformative, and I am confident that it will bring positive changes to your life.

If you found this book helpful, I kindly ask you to leave a review or share it with others who could benefit from the information. Your feedback and support will help spread the message of self-care and aromatherapy to a wider audience.

Thank you once again for joining me on this journey. I wish you continued success and well-being in all aspects of your life.

GLOSSARY

Absorption: The process by which essential oils are taken into the body or absorbed by the skin.

Analgesic: A substance that helps relieve pain and reduce discomfort. Essential oils with analgesic properties have soothing and pain-relieving effects when applied topically or inhaled.

Antimicrobial: The ability of a substance or agent to inhibit the growth or kill microorganisms such as bacteria, viruses, fungi, or other pathogens. Essential oils with antimicrobial properties can help reduce the presence of harmful microorganisms and promote a cleaner and healthier environment.

Antiseptic: An essential oil that possesses properties that help prevent the growth of microorganisms and inhibit infections.

Aromatherapy: The use of essential oils with the aim of improving one's physical, mental, and emotional health.

Blend: A combination of two or more essential oils mixed together to create a desired fragrance or therapeutic effect.

Calming: Essential oils are known for their soothing and relaxing properties and are often used to promote a sense of tranquility and reduce stress.

Carrier oil: To dilute essential oils for topical use, a neutral base oil is employed.

Cleansing: Essential oils with purifying properties are often used in cleaning products or for detoxifying the body.

Cold pressing: A common technique for mechanically extracting essential oils from citrus fruits.

Diffuser: A tool that spreads essential oils in the air, enabling them to be inhaled for the purpose of aromatherapy.

Dilution: Diluting essential oils involves mixing them with a carrier oil or another material that is compatible with them. This helps prevent any adverse effects.

Distillation: The most common method of extracting essential oils; involves the separation of volatile compounds from plant material through steam or water.

Energizing: Essential oils that have stimulating and invigorating effects are often used to combat fatigue and promote alertness.

Essential oil: Highly concentrated plant extracts obtained through various extraction methods, containing the volatile aromatic compounds of plants.

Eucalyptol: A compound found in eucalyptus essential oil known for its expectorant and decongestant properties.

Expectorant: Essential oils that help to loosen and expel mucus from the respiratory system, aiding in relief from congestion and coughs.

Extraction: The process of obtaining essential oils from plant material, which can include methods like steam distillation, cold pressing, or solvent extraction.

Floral: A category of essential oils derived from flowers, often characterized by their sweet, delicate, and romantic scents.

Grounding: Essential oils with established grounding and stabilizing characteristics are used to encourage equilibrium and emotional steadiness.

Hydrosol: Also known as floral water or herbal distillate, it is the aromatic water that remains after the distillation of essential oils.

Immune support: Essential oils that have properties believed to strengthen and support the immune system.

Inhalation: The method of using essential oils by breathing in their aroma, often through diffusers or inhalers, for their therapeutic effects.

Nervine: Essential oils known for their calming and soothing effects on the nervous system are often used to relieve anxiety and promote relaxation.

Patch test: A method of testing a small amount of diluted essential oil on a small area of the skin to check for any adverse reactions.

Resin: A type of essential oil derived from the resinous sap or gum of certain trees, known for their rich, warm, and balsamic aromas.

Roller blend: A roller blend is a mixture of essential oils diluted in a carrier oil and stored in a roller bottle for easy and controlled application to the skin. It allows for the targeted and convenient use of essential oils for various purposes, such as aromatherapy and personal care. The rollerball top on the bottle ensures smooth and precise application.

Sensitization: A reaction that can occur when an individual develops an allergic response to a particular essential oil after repeated exposure.

Shelf life: The period during which an essential oil is considered stable and retains its therapeutic properties when stored properly.

Solubility: The ability of an essential oil to dissolve or mix with another substance, such as water or carrier oils.

Solvent extraction: An extraction method that involves using a solvent, such as hexane, to dissolve the essential oil from the plant material.

Synergy: The combined effect of two or more essential oils working together to enhance their individual properties.

Therapeutic grade: A term used to describe essential oils that are believed to meet specific quality and purity standards for therapeutic use.

Tonic: Essential oils that have a strengthening and invigorating effect on the body and mind are often used to promote overall wellness.

Topical application: The practice of applying diluted essential oils directly to the skin for absorption and localized benefits.

Uplifting: Essential oils known for their mood-enhancing properties are often used to uplift spirits and promote a positive outlook.

Volatile: This refers to the characteristic of essential oils to evaporate or vaporize easily at normal temperatures, releasing their aroma into the air.

REFERENCES

A Comprehensive Guide to Essential Oil Extraction Methods. (2017). Newdirectionsaromatics.com. https://www.newdirectionsaromatics.com/blog/articles/how-essential-oils-are-made.html

Agero, A. L. C., & Verallo-Rowell, V. M. (2004). *A Randomized Double-Blind Controlled Trial Comparing Extra Virgin Coconut Oil with Mineral Oil as a Moisturizer for Mild to Moderate Xerosis.* Dermatitis (Formerly American Journal of Contact Dermatitis), 15(03), 109. https://pubmed.ncbi.nlm.nih.gov/15724344/

Anderson, E. (2020, August 17). *Essential Oils – An Overview.* Center for Research on Ingredient Safety. https://www.canr.msu.edu/news/essential-oils-an-overview

Anglis, J. (2019, September 26). *7 Celebrities Who Use Essential Oils.* First for Women. https://www.firstforwomen.com/gallery/entertainment/celebrities-who-use-essential-oils-172818

Axe, J. (2022, January 28). *What Are the Best Carrier Oils?* Dr. Axe. https://draxe.com/essential-oils/carrier-oils-for-essential-oils/

Ballard, C. G., O'Brien, J. T., Reichelt, K., & Perry, E. K. (2002). *Aromatherapy as a Safe and Effective Treatment for the Management of Agitation in Severe Dementia: The Results of a Double-Blind, Placebo-Controlled Trial with Melissa.* The Journal of clinical psychiatry, 63(7), 553–558. https://doi.org/10.4088/jcp.v63n0703

Barton, N. (2018, November 22). *Essential Oils for Breaking Bad Habits and Addictive Behaviour.* Retrieved June 1, 2023, from www.baseformula.com. https://www.baseformula.com/blog/essential-oils-for-cravings-addiction

Bethesda. (2002). *PDQ Cancer Information Summaries.* In PubMed. National Cancer Institute (US). https://www.ncbi.nlm.nih.gov/books/NBK82221/

Blair, C. (2020, January 7). *Are Essential Oils Safe for Children?* www.hopkinsallchildrens.org. https://www.hopkinsallchildrens.org/ACH-News/General-News/Are-Essential-Oils-Safe-for-Children

Buerger, M. (2019, December 11). *Essential oils are potent, risky and promising. Here's what you need to know.* Washington Post. https://www.washingtonpost.com/lifestyle/wellness/essential-oils-are-potent-risky-and-promis ing-heres-what-you-need-to-know/2019/12/10/1470d7c4-1623-11ea-8406-df3c54b3253e_story.html.

Capritto, A. (2020, November 4). *The dangers of essential oils: Why natural isn't always safe.* CNET. https://www.cnet.com/health/are-essential-oils-actually-safe/

Carter, E. (2022, June 14). *15 DIY Massage Oil Recipes for All Occasions – Using Essential Oils.* Essential Oil Haven. https://www.essentialoilhaven.com/diy-massage-oil-recipes/

CDC: Sleep and Sleep Disorders. (2023). Centers for Disease Control and Prevention. Retrieved June 1, 2023, from https://www.cdc.gov/sleep/index.html

Charlotte. (2020, December 30). How Hormones Affect Energy Levels. *BodyLogicMD.* Retrieved June 1, 2023, from https://www.bodylogicmd.com/blog/how-hormones-affect-energy-levels/

Christine. (2019, March 1). *Essential Oil Dilution Chart, Calculator & Ratio Guide.* www.mountainroseherbs.com. Retrieved June 1, 2023, from https://blog.mountainroseherbs.com/essential-oil-dilutions

Davis, B. (2023, April 11). *Limonene Terpene.* The Konnexion. Thekonnexion.com. https://thekonnexion.com/limonene-terpene/

Del Carmen Hernandez, M. (2021, December 22). 10 Benefits of Essential Oils for Babies and Children. *You Are Mom.* https://youaremom.com/children/what-should-you-know/tips-for-raising-your-child/essential-oils/

Dessinger, H. (2016, March 21). Safe Essential Oils For Pregnancy and Breastfeeding. *Mommypotamus.* https://mommypotamus.com/essential-oils-pregnancy/

Dessinger, H. (2021, May 29). *Which Essential Oils Are Safe For Kids? 70+ Oils & How To Use Them.* Mommypotamus. https://mommypotamus.com/safe-essential-oils-babies-children/

Ellis, L. (2022, August 4). What Perfume Does Ellen Pompeo Wear? *Celeb Answers.* Retrieved May 30, 2023, from https://celebanswers.com/what-perfume-does-ellen-pompeo-wear/

Enshaieh, S., Jooya, A., Siadat, A. H., & Iraji, F. (2007). The efficacy of 5% topical tea tree oil gel in mild to moderate acne vulgaris: a randomized, double-blind placebo-controlled study. *Indian Journal Of Dermatology, Venereology And Leprology*, 73(1), 22–25. https://doi.org/10.4103/0378-6323.30646

Essential Oils. (n.d.). National Institute of Environmental Health Sciences.

Retrieved June 1, 2023, from https://www.niehs.nih.gov/health/topics/agents/essential-oils/index.cfm

Essential Oils Handbook Quotes by Amy Leigh Mercree. (2023). Goodreads.com. https://www.goodreads.com/work/quotes/58054493-essential-oils-hand book-recipes-for-natural-living-volume-2

FDA: Aromatherapy. (2022). *U.S. Food and Drug Administration*. Retrieved on June 30, 2023 from https://www.fda.gov/cosmetics/cosmetic-products/aromatherapy

FDA: Is It a Cosmetic, a Drug, or Both? (Or Is It Soap?). (2022). *U.S. Food and Drug Administration*. https://www.fda.gov/cosmetics/cosmetics-laws-regu lations/it-cosmetic-drug-or-both-or-it-soap#:~:text=The%20Federal% 20Food%2C%20Drug%2C%20and%20Cosmetic%20Act%20%28FD%26C

Feel handsome, smell awesome: 7 essential oils for men. (2019, November 4). *Young Living Blog*. https://www.youngliving.com/blog/essential-oils-for-men/

Fisher, K. and Phillips, C.A. (2006), The effect of lemon, orange and bergamot essential oils and their components on the survival of Campylobacter jejuni, Escherichia coli O157, Listeria monocytogenes, Bacillus cereus and Staphylococcus aureus in vitro and in food systems. *Journal of Applied Microbiology*, 101: 1232-1240. https://doi.org/10.1111/j.1365-2672.2006.03035.x

Fokou, J. B. H., Dongmo, P. M. J., & Boyom, F. F. (2020). Essential oil's chem ical composition and pharmacological properties. In *IntechOpen*. https://www.intechopen.com/chapters/68008

Frothingham, S. (2019, August 20). *18 essential oils you can use to boost your energy*. Healthline. Retrieved May 30, 2023, from https://www.healthline.com/health/essential-oils-for-energy#5-backed-by-research

Galper, A., & Shutes, J. (2020, October 11). *The ultimate guide to aromatherapy: an illustrated guide to blending essential oils and crafting remedies for body, mind, and spirit*. Barnes & Noble. https://www.barnesandnoble.com/w/the-ultimate-guide-to-aromatherapy-jade-shutes/1137661119

Halcon, L. (n.d.). *Are Essential Oils Safe? Taking Charge of Your Health & Wellbe ing*. Retrieved July 6, 2023, from https://www.takingcharge.csh.umn.edu/are-essential-oils-safe

Harper, E. (2016, July 1). *Safe essential oils for babies and how to use them*. Health line. Retrieved May 31, 2023, from https://www.healthline.com/health/parenting/essential-oils-for-babies

Harvard School of Public Health. (2021, April). *Cravings.* The Nutrition Source. https://www.hsph.harvard.edu/nutritionsource/cravings/

Hay, I. C., Jamieson, M., & Ormerod, A. D. (1998). Randomized trial of aromatherapy. Successful treatment for alopecia areata. *Archives of Dermatology,* 134(11), 1349–1352. https://doi.org/10.1001/archderm.134.11.1349

Heather. (2017, January 11). Everything You Need to Know about Grades of Essential Oils. *A Real Food Journey.* https://www.arealfoodjourney.com/grades-of-essential-oils/

How do I determine the quality of essential oils? Taking charge of your health & wellbeing. (n.d.). Taking Charge of Your Health & Wellbeing. https://www.takingcharge.csh.umn.edu/how-do-i-determine-quality-essential-oils

Homemade Cucumber Mandarin Face Mask with Essential Oils. (2016, May 19). Encouraging Moms at Home. https://encouragingmomsathome.com/homemade-cucumber-mandarin-face-mask-essential-oils/

How your hormones affect your energy levels. (2023). Thriva Health Hub. Retrieved May 31, 2023, from https://thriva.co/hub/womens-health/how-your-hormones-affect-your-energy-levels

Johnson, J. (2019, October 18). *Everything you need to know about essential oils.* Medical News Today. Retrieved May 31, 2023, from https://www.medicalnewstoday.com/articles/326732

Khare, V. (2018, March 26). 6 Foods To Eat To Gain Weight And Mass. *Be Beautiful India.* Retrieved June 22, 2023, from https://www.bebeautiful.in/articles/6-foods-to-eat-to-gain-weight-and-mass

Lane, J. (2022, November 17). What are the best essential oils for massage? *Loving Essential Oils.* Retrieved May 20, 2023, from www.lovingessentialoils.com. https://www.lovingessentialoils.com/blogs/aromatherapy-news/what-are-the-best-essential-oils-for-massage

Mahdavikian, S., Rezaei, M., Modarresi, M., & Khatony, A. (2020). Comparing the effect of aromatherapy with peppermint and lavender on the sleep quality of cardiac patients: a randomized controlled trial. *Sleep Science and Practice,* 4(1). https://doi.org/10.1186/s41606-020-00047-x

Martinez, B. (2022, May 5). Is there a grading system for essential oils?- AAA. *Edens Garden.* https://www.edensgarden.com/blogs/news/is-there-a-grading-system-for-essential-oils-aaa

McDermott, A. (2017, August 15). *How to use carrier oils.* Healthline. https://www.healthline.com/health/carrier-oil

Mizrahi, B., Shapira, L., Domb, A. J., & Houri-Haddad, Y. (2006). Citrus oil and MgCl2 as antibacterial and anti-inflammatory agents. *Journal of Periodontology*, 77(6), 963–968. https://doi.org/10.1902/jop.2006.050278

NCCIH: Aromatherapy. (2020, January). NCCIH. https://www.nccih.nih.gov/health/aromatherapy

Nelson, N. (2013, October 14). *Homemade Shampoo with Essential Oils*. Tiny Apothecary. https://shalommama.com/homemade-shampoo

Nervik, T. (2021, February 28). What is Aromatherapy and Essential Oils? *Volant Europe*. Retrieved May 23, 2023, from https://volantaroma.com/blogs/guides/what-is-aromatherapy-and-essential-oils

Neville, L. (2022, May 10). Estrogen, Progesterone And Thyroid Hormones: Friends Or Foes? Dr. Laura Neville. https://doctorneville.com/blog/2022/5/5/estrogen-progestone-and-thyroid-hormones-friends-or-foes

Pace, S. (2019, February 8). *Essential oils in hospitals: the ethics, safety, cost and application of clinical aromatherapy*. Tisserand Institute. https://tisserandinstitute.org/essential-oils-in-hospitals/

Petruzzi, D. (2022, February 16). *Topic: Essential Oils*. www.statista.com. https://www.statista.com/topics/5174/essential-oils/

Practical use of essential oils. (2023). London Acupuncture at Cure by Nature. https://cure-by-nature.co.uk/London%20homeopathy/essential%20oils/

Purdie, J. (2016, October 17). *Best Essential Oils for Weight Loss?* Healthline. https://www.healthline.com/health/diet-and-weight-loss/essential-oils-for-weight-loss

Quality & Grades of Essential Oils. (2020, February 12). Nature's Lab. https://natureslab.com/blogs/news/quality-grades-of-essential-oils

Stierwalt, S. (2020, March 7). *Do Essential Oils Work? Here's What Science Says*. Scientific American. Retrieved June 1, 2023, from https://www.scientificamerican.com/article/do-essential-oils-work-heres-what-science-says/

Sullivan, D. (2023, April 10). 19+ Amazing essential oils that promote weight loss. *Native American Nutritionals*. Retrieved June 1, 2023, from https://gyalabs.com/blogs/essential-oils/best-essential-oils-for-weight-loss

Sweeney, M. (2020, August 20). *Do essential oils expire?* Healthline. Retrieved June 1, 2023, from https://www.healthline.com/health/do-essential-oils-expire#average-shelf-life

The regulatory landscape of essential oil manufacturing navigating FDA and international regulations. (2023, May 10). Vriaroma.com. https://vriaroma.

com/blog/106/the-regulatory-landscape-of-essential-oil-manufacturing-navigating-fda-and-international-regulations

Tomaino, J. (n.d.). *FDA Regulation of essential oils - what do I need to know about safety and quality?* Coursera. Retrieved June 6, 2023, from https://www. coursera.org/lecture/aromatherapy-clinical-use-essential-oils/fda-regula tion-of-essential-oils-1eBtI

20 Best Homemade Laundry Detergent. (2023, June 2). *News Direct Corp.* https://www.newsdirect.com/home-goods/best-homemade-laundry-detergent

Villafranco, S. (2018, April 15). *How to make essential oils.* Mindbodygreen. https://www.mindbodygreen.com/articles/how-essential-oils-are-made

Watson, K., Hatcher, D., & Good, A. (2019). A randomised controlled trial of Lavender (Lavandula Angustifolia) and Lemon Balm (Melissa Officinalis) essential oils for the treatment of agitated behaviour in older people with and without dementia. *Complementary Therapies in Medicine*, 42, 366–373. https://doi.org/10.1016/j.ctim.2018.12.016

West, H. (2019, September 30). *What are essential oils, and do they work?* Health-line. Retrieved May 31, 2023, from https://www.healthline.com/nutri tion/what-are-essential-oils

Wohlner, O. (2020, December 11). *Kerry Washington's Three-Ingredient Scalp Spray is 'Walking Aromatherapy'.* NewBeauty. Retrieved May 30, 2023, from https://www.newbeauty.com/kerry-washington-scalp-spray/

IMAGE REFERENCES

Bright, K. (2019, December 7). *Make-up brush photo* [Images]. Unsplash. https://unsplash.com/photos/drRdk8BI43Q

Chamara, PMV (2021, September 11) *A group of purple bottles sitting on top of a table photo* [Images]. Unsplash. https://unsplash.com/photos/ OXYOFT9gTOE

DoTerra International, LLC. (2019, May 15). *Woman smelling a bottle of essen-tial oil* [Image]. Pexels. https://www.pexels.com/photo/woman-smelling-a-bottle-of-essential-oil-3969195/

Mathews, S. (2023, June 23). *Best oils* [Image]. Canva. www.canva.com

Mathews, S. (2023, June 23). *Label design* [Image]. Canva. www.canva.com

Mikan, L. (2018, May 14). *Woman sitting with baby on her lap surrounded with purple flowers* [Images]. Unsplash. https://unsplash.com/photos/6KRmH6k3Rdk

Pixabay. (2016, February 16). *Books in black wooden bookshelf* [Images]. Pexels. https://www.pexels.com/photo/books-in-black-wooden-book-shelf-159711/

Sang-ngern, P. (2019, January 19). *Crop women with decorative heart sitting near child* [Images]. Pexels. https://www.pexels.com/photo/crop-women-with-decorative-hearts-sitting-near-child-5340266/

Schneider, P. (2016, October 6) *Light bulbs and vines* [Images]. Unsplash. https://unsplash.com/photos/mFnbFaCIu1I.

Seegars, K. (2020, December 21). *Person holding brown and white cup* [Images]. Unsplash. https://unsplash.com/photos/v1ZT8Y76hqc

Shapouri, C. (2019, May 2). *Votive candle photo* [Image]. Unsplash. https://unsplash.com/photos/r40EYKVyutI

Sikkema, K. (2017, December 10). *Essential oils at home* [Images]. Unsplash. https://unsplash.com/photos/UaO58q6ioxI

Volant (2021, November 12). *Grey volant diffuser and essential oils add ambiance and transform the kitchen into a relaxing environment* [Images]. Unsplash. https://unsplash.com/photos/1aKZ5tVygKE

Thank you for reading Aromatherapy for Self Care. Click on the QR Code below for your FREE 21 Essential Oil Guide

Made in the USA
Middletown, DE
14 October 2023

40606790R00116